What People Are Saying About *Beyond Belief*

"In a world that seeks to avoid suffering at all costs (certainly an impossible goal) Kyle Campbell leads us on a journey to embrace suffering as a means for discovering one's purpose. This counterintuitive approach to life is honest, real, and ultimately hopeful. We discover through Kyle's story of living life with a rare brain stem tumor that suffering is normative to the human condition and pursuing the 'why' of suffering leads to a deadend street. His reflections as to how God uses suffering to shape us into the persons God wants us to become are surprising, biblical, Jesus-centered, and full of ancient wisdom.

If you suffer, and all people eventually do, read this book to trade in your 'why questions' for the better path of growth, purpose, and joy through God's redemptive work in and through suffering. Kyle shows us the way."

—Charles Revis, D. Min.
Executive Minister, Mission Northwest

"Kyle Campbell has authored an exceptional book that brings deeper meaning in pursuing our faith and purpose in life. He opens our eyes to the medical aspects of disability and the human experience in transcending life's barriers to move forward and focus on the question: ***Now what?***

Campbell challenges us to avoid the 'why me' question and answer to a higher calling:

'Each day we are alive, that is one less day we have to live on Earth, one less day to build a legacy, to leave an

impact. How do we spend our time? Does it align with our values? More importantly, does it align with God's values? When asked to give an account of our lives, what are we going to say?'

Kyle provides the tools to help us answer these questions and many more. No matter what season of life you are in, this book was written for you."

—Dr. Steven Koobatian
President, Vocational Designs, Inc.
Faculty, California State University, Fresno

"If you are struggling now with any kind of physical disability, this book is a ***must-read*** for you! Kyle's testimony of how he overcame his disability will inspire you to carry on and most of all to turn to God and Jesus Christ to help you adapt and overcome your disability!

I have known Kyle all his life. I have seen and heard about all his struggles over the years starting with the fireplace burn, then his brain stem tumor, and many others. In reading his book I am amazed by how Kyle has adapted and survived his many physical and emotional challenges.

Most of all I admire Kyle for moving from trying to figure everything out with logic to relying on and trusting God and Jesus Christ to strengthen him and lead him."

—Patrick Montgomery, PhD

"Kyle has opened up my eyes and my heart to my own personal and spiritual struggles. His book answered the questions I've fought for many years to answer. Kyle's inspiring experiences allowed me to see through my own son's lens and past his disability. It is a book I wish to gift to my son when he gets older so that he can overcome the barriers and obstacles of his disability through hope and the knowledge that anything is possible with God!

This book is fascinating, informative, and suspenseful. A perfect resource for just about anything, but most importantly, for anyone looking for hope. Kyle is living proof that God keeps his promises and God promises that he will never leave us nor forsake us."

—Yee Z. Lee

"*Beyond Belief* is an uplifting account of determination, grit, and overcoming overwhelming odds. Kyle Campbell speaks directly to his experiences of living with an inoperable brain tumor, but his story doesn't just apply to those with a similar diagnosis. No matter what you are facing in life, Kyle's faith, hope, and perseverance are sure to inspire you. His story tangibly proves the hope found in Jesus, a hope that is available to everyone!"

—Melissa Moore
On-Air Radio Host, Spirit Radio in Visalia

"*Beyond Belief* is Kyle Campbell's vivid account of dealing with the disability and treatment of a brain tumor which was diagnosed when he was five years old. Kyle tells his story in a straightforward, almost matter of fact style. It reflects the growing spiritual maturity of Kyle and his family and their willingness to submit to the medical protocols of world-class physicians, and to trust Christ.

Jesus' spirit is reflected in Kyle and in his book. This is a book about what Christ can do in a life surrendered to him. Read it and give it to the person you know who needs help and hope to deal with a chronic illness, a failing marriage, or other catastrophe. Kyle's testimony in *Beyond Belief* will encourage them."

—Harry Wood
Pastor Emeritus, Visalia Methodist Church

"Kyle has given a direct look into living life, not only with a disability, but also living the best life with the Lord Jesus Christ. Anyone who reads this book will be challenged to live life to his or her full potential. Kyle has inspired me to an even greater desire to live daily with joy. In this book, he offers insightful ideas on how anyone can start living that life today!

I have known Kyle since he was a newborn and his family is dear to my heart. My wife and I were honored to have him as our ring bearer in our wedding. As Kyle was healing from the awful burn to his left hand, I was recovering from an almost fatal motorcycle accident which left my arm paralyzed. Like Kyle, I have struggled, but that wasn't the end of the narrative. I now live with a permanent disability, but have overcome it with my Savior. Having experienced my own life-altering events, Kyle's book really hit home with me. And I too, can truly say that with God, all things are possible!"

—Jeffrey S. Ellis, MA Theology
Pastor, Landmark Missionary Baptist Church

BEYOND
Belief

How Living with a Brain Stem Tumor Brought
Faith and **Purpose** to **Life**

KYLE CAMPBELL

Publishing support provided by
Ignite Press
5070 N. Sixth St. #189
Fresno, CA 93710
www.IgnitePress.us

ISBN: 979-8-9868142-0-9
ISBN: 979-8-9868142-1-6 (Ebook)

For bulk purchase and for booking, contact:

Kyle Campbell
Kyle.BeyondBelief@gmail.com
www.KyleBeyondBelief.com

Library of Congress Control Number: 2022914625

Cover design by Usman Tariq
Edited by Charlie Wormhoudt
Interior design by Eswari Kamireddy

FIRST EDITION

F1

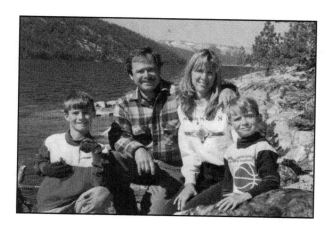

This book is dedicated to my family: my mom (Marcia), my dad (Gary), and my brother (Tyler). In this photo Tyler is on the left, holding lizards. I'm the little guy on the right. We have all been through this medical journey together. A lot of it is not just my story, it's our story. Thank you Mom and Dad, for helping me develop the perspective to recognize each day as a gift, and to celebrate the small victories. Thank you Tyler, for being my brother and my friend growing up—someone who was always there to do fun, regular kid stuff with (like catching lizards). Thank you also to Nana, and to all the friends and family who joined us through this journey. Your support and prayers have been monumental.

This book is dedicated to people with brain tumors (and their families, who are also on the journey with us). You are so resilient, whether you're a survivor (like me) or still living with your tumor (like me). It's a part of life, and our tumors can often become tied to our identities. Our impairments and symptoms can go up or down in severity throughout the day, but they are always there, when we wake up and go to bed. Our brain tumors can be frustrating and scary, and *they can also be a blessing—which might sound crazy to someone without a brain tumor, but if you are in the Gray Club (tumors on MRIs appear in a light gray color) I have a hunch you know what I'm talking about.*

This book, lastly, is dedicated to people who do not survive their brain tumors. They are not forgotten and did not spend their lives in vain. Thank you for the legacy you've left for us, for your families, and for society.

Acknowledgments

This book wouldn't have been written if I wasn't here. Thank you to my care team and all the doctors, nurses, technicians, and medical staff who have treated or assisted me in treatment. I wouldn't be here without all of you. I doubt all of you will see this, but I appreciate you all.

This book wouldn't be what it is without the editorial support of Andrew Luis and Patrick Montgomery. Your suggestions were instrumental in my telling of this story. Also, thank you to Kelsey Luis, Steve Koobatian, Melissa Moore, Pastor Jeff Ellis, Pastor Charles Revis, Pastor Harry Wood, Bill Yoshimoto, Yee Lee, and all other readers and contributors. It's a gift to be able to share this story, and you all have taken part in that opportunity.

A special thanks to my amazing wife, Lori, for her faithful encouragement and unwavering support in this book project.

Finally, thanks to the team at Ignite Press for helping me put this book together into an engaging format and design. Much has been added to this project with their expertise and guidance.

CONTENTS

Introduction

Hello, my name is Kyle, and I'm really excited to write this book. It can seem daunting to write a book, and a million things can keep someone from writing things down. I actually started writing this ten years ago, but I had no direction back then. I just knew I had to share my story, but I didn't know how at that time.

When you have a story to tell that impacts your life to the extent mine has, there is no keeping it contained. And I'm so thankful that I've finally learned how to tell this story.

I'm looking forward to sharing my journey of living, striving, and thriving through a childhood brain stem tumor, radiation treatment, and more. My goal is to inspire hope and perspective in someone with a similar (and maybe recent) diagnosis, their family, their friends, or anyone who may be experiencing various challenges in life.

Through sharing my struggles, successes, and ongoing symptoms through daily life, my goal is that people might replace feelings of loneliness with belonging, discouragement with hope, and helplessness with empowerment. I share my story freely and invite you to do with it what you will. After all, my story isn't about me—it's about you.

Why did I call this book Beyond Belief?

I had difficulty coming up with a title for this book, and changed it probably four times. I'm going with *Beyond Belief* for several reasons:

The first is the definition of *beyond belief* having to do with something extraordinary, something so uncommon it's hard to believe at first. I believe my story meets that definition. To me, my story is totally normal. I've grown up with it and have never known anything else. I don't know what it's like to *not* have a brain tumor. But I've noticed whenever I tell people who know me what I've been through, they're usually shocked and it takes a minute for the story to sink in. For those people, they might say my story is *beyond belief.*

Another reason, and the primary reason, I went with *Beyond Belief* is more philosophical. I think absolute knowledge is real and out there, but beyond our grasp at certain times. For those things beyond our limits for knowledge we have belief. We believe all sorts of things: science, religion, global warming, various theories, that Star Wars is an amazing story of the redemption of Anakin Skywalker, that *Star Trek: The Original Series* is the best series . . . We believe SO many things. Some of our beliefs are extremely well founded and supported by an overwhelming amount of evidence (global warming, for example) while other beliefs are less supported by evidence and may be more subjective to the individual (whether *The Original Series* is the best series of Star Trek).

When we move *beyond belief,* we are taking a belief and making it *personal* through conviction. We are taking our personal confidence in a belief and assigning an action to it.

This book is about the action of conviction through faith. And this conviction for me, this story, came to be fueled through my medical challenges.

I was three years old when I had my first medical scare. I severely burned my left hand. I was excitedly running around the house when I tripped near the fireplace and my left hand shot in. I screamed out in pain as my hand touched the metal grate holding the burning logs of our roaring fire. When I tried to pull my hand out, it got lodged between the safety screen and the bottom of the fireplace. After rapidly pulling out my hand, my parents put it under some cool water and rushed me to the hospital in their car, my mom singing "Rudolph, the Red-Nosed Reindeer" to keep me calm. My third-degree burn landed me in the burn unit. I was hospitalized for a while, my parents taking turns staying with their three-year-old. After my burn treatments and surgery, I made it home in time for Christmas wearing a cast. And I got to keep all my fingers! I had to wear a protective glove for a few years. I have quite the scar, and have had several skin graft surgeries since then.

This book is actually inspired by my other major medical journey, which is still very much ongoing. I was diagnosed with a brain stem tumor at five years old, and I still have it. I've been living, striving, and thriving with this thing my whole life. There have been times of challenge, and there have been times of joy.

I can count on one hand the number of people I've met who also have had a brain tumor, and I can count on half of those fingers the people who have survived. When I look for books people have written about having brain tumors, I find a handful of accounts—but I haven't seen one yet about a brain stem tumor. The only brain stem tumor books I found were for doctors, written by other doctors. Surviving and living with a brain stem tumor is an incredible blessing, as well as a challenge. I've journeyed from a grim, "The prognosis is *not* good . . . " at age five, to thriving 30 years later.

I've earned a bachelor's degree in philosophy from Cal Poly San Luis Obispo (with an emphasis in epistemology and the difference between knowledge and belief), a master's degree in rehabilitation counseling from California State University, Fresno, and hold national certification as a Certified Rehabilitation Counselor. Currently, I'm employed at a community college working in student services. There, I help people with various disabilities matriculate into college and navigate through their studies.

I am a Christian, a husband, a father, a son, a brother, and a friend. I am a Star Wars, Lord of the Rings, and Marvel Studios fan. I have been a preacher, a professor, and a poet.

Another thing to know about me is that I love stories—telling, listening to, and sharing them. I like getting caught up in characters and different peoples' perspectives. Understanding why somebody else does what they decide to do can be fascinating. We gain so much from sharing stories; they have the power to influence a decision, make someone smile, and even change a life.

When I talk about stories, I'm not thinking about the ones we make up for fun. I enjoy those fictional stories—especially Westerns where the good guys always get the bad guys in the end. But when I say I love stories, I'm referring to perspectives based on personal experience. Stories are based on challenges faced as individuals and what we learn from those challenges—what we gain from our experiences. I'm talking about personal testimony.

We all have so many amazing things to share because we all have different struggles, trials, and challenges that we go through. The challenges we experience can either leave us feeling defeated, or they can teach us great things we would never have learned otherwise. We all are capable of sharing our wisdom. Some of us have more wisdom than others (based on what we do with our experiences), but we all have something. We all have so much we can share. It is a duty, and a privilege, to be able to share those things.

I was embarrassed about my story for so long, and, at times, even ashamed of it. It made me different from everybody else. Parts of my story made me not who I wanted to be. I wanted to be the same as everyone else because that's what you think is good when you're a kid. My challenges, I believe, made me grow up pretty fast. I learned how great it is to be different. And what makes me different is my story and what I've learned throughout this life.

This book has four parts: Part One is about my medical journey and struggle; Part Two is about faith and philosophy; Part Three is about development and emotion; and Part Four is about **you** and how **you** might move forward after having read this book. In Part Four, I'll share with you some of the life lessons I have learned about how to intentionally live a hopeful, joy-filled, and meaningful life.

Before sharing my journey, I want to set the tone of this book with a poem I wrote in 2012, in the midst of my transformation.

Discovery:
A Poem of Transformation

It was the quietest part of the night as I hunched over the keyboard, not knowing what I was going to write . . . but knowing, *beyond belief*, that I needed to write something. It was my valley of the shadow of death, the point where life is hardest. This wasn't how life was supposed to go. Something had to *and was going to* change. This poem is what God gave to me in that moment.

A Lesson to be Learned

Bad things happen for good reasons.
Although it blinds and divides,
change is in the season.
The time for fun and games is done.
There are rivers to be swum, mountains to be clumb,
valleys to be crossed, and battles to be won.

Boom! The lightning screams as you're shocked out of sleep.
There are no clouds in the sky. There is no rain falling down.
The slope you descend becomes steep.
You tumble past the trees, *whish* and *whoosh*!
Past the trees standing so stably with their deep roots,
you land with a *thump*, dazed and confused.

Dazed and confused, you glance around,
attempt to get your bearings,
but then fail with a frown.
It is too dark to see, too much to bear.
A prickly tingle goes up your back
and you realize you can't go anywhere.

Lost and lonely, you sweat in desperation.
If only you knew which way to go,
which way to face, or your general location
you might find help; you might become found.
But then you remember the creeping darkness,
and all of your hopes vanish into the ground.

This fall takes you back to a notch in your clock
when dark things reigned in your life
and you couldn't wait for that next *tock*.
You try to remember, "Oh, what did I do?
How did I survive? How did I escape
that moment I was feeling so blue?"

Reaching and grasping, running and roaming,
ducking and diving through the dark stormy gloom,
you stop moving to think . . . and thank God for remembering!
"How does one deal with stormy situations?"
You batten up the hatches!
And prepare the preparations!

And what do the preparations include?
They include a code to live by,
a God at your side, and an attitude that can-do.
Because what makes it easy to feel lost in defeat?

Ignorance, doubt, fear, stress,
and a lonely feeling with no one to greet.

Goodness keeps your mind at ease,
as your instincts say to hide and flee.
Self-control brings you to peace
as your gut-feeling shouts, "Panic! Cry!"
Perseverance makes you strong at heart
as the world tells you just to lay down and die.

But wait! What's that at your feet?
As you fall to the floor and feel a great roar,
you can maybe, almost, just barely see, though vague and discreet,
a light, far away, as a candle freshly put out.
There is only a faint glow,
but enough to bring hope. You give out a shout!

You wander toward the light,
tripping and falling among the roots and rocks.
Could this bring salvation? It just might!
Faster and faster, brighter and brighter,
the light draws near,
as your feet become lighter.

"Freedom!" you exclaim as you enter a meadow
with bright sunshine falling over where the green grass grows,
where the trees grow tall and the blue waters flow.
Beauty, magnificence, awe, and splendor;
where did this come from?
You look around and ponder in wonder.

Surely, this place is better than before.

Though the tumble down was long and dark,
you're beginning to be grateful, more and more,
for the dark road you were forced to go down,
for, eventually, it led to something good.
Though it had you scared stiff, you came to be found.

Found! As the light becomes day
and the day shines so bright,
you wonder how you ever found the way
out of that dark and lonely place,
where bad things happen
and evil shows its face.

There is no mountain without a valley.
There is no rise without a fall.
Look around at the gloom, and think of how it could be.
It could be peaceful, a place that's serene.
Like coming to a breathtaking meadow from the empty dark,
we must only have faith in what is unseen.

And stay holding on, just a little longer, we must.
Before our bones turn to ashes
or our dreams start to rust.
For if we sustain darkness and persevere through the test,
we just might find the light,
and discover our journey was for the best.

But do not go unarmed; do not go alone!
For long is the journey
and dark is the road.
Do not trust appearances; you are only half.
There is another you must take;

He bears a rod and staff.

His rod and staff will comfort you
as the darkness creeps and leads to folly.
Some of his strength He will imbue
if only you declare and claim.
You will find joy in the journey
and, in the painful, not so much pain.

Will you be lost in the forest and get out on your own?
Maybe. But if the present reflects the past,
then your chances are blown.
So choose your side! Take the dare!
But if you do, make sure you do.
Not for me, but for you. Anytime! Anywhere!

PART 1:

Journey and Healing

Heartbreak

After graduating from college, I worked in a group home for teenagers for three years. These kids were labeled "at-risk" youth, meaning that there was a high potential for them to end up in gangs, on the streets, homeless, or on drugs. These were kids without families or kids from families needing extra support raising them.

One day, I attended a conference convened around the topic of gang violence. It was early morning, and the event was just getting started. I had never been to a conference before and was excited to learn what these people had to say about life. Their speech actually started with a story about death. Two fathers were talking about gang prevention that day. One father's son had killed the other father's son in an act of gang violence. Now, the two were doing conferences together to help prevent kids from getting caught up in gang violence. Typically, death follows life. Here was a time when Death inspired new Life.

The main speakers of the event that day had a quote to share, and it went like this:

"God will break your heart, over and over again, until it will finally stay open."

There are many ways to experience a broken heart: family problems, financial situations, relationships going south, and more. All sorts of things can tear us apart inside.

I didn't realize at the time how much this message would prove true in my life.

Diagnosis

When I was five years old, my mom noticed things about me that were unusual and did not quite reflect normal child development. I had a super high-pitched voice with lots of nasality in my speech. My parents took me to a doctor to see if everything was okay. The first doctor we went to told us, "Yeah, he's fine; he's just developing his speech slower, and he'll be okay—give him time."

My mom was unsatisfied with that answer. She wanted a second opinion to make sure that nothing was going on. The second doctor thought maybe I should be taken to a neurologist, that perhaps something was going on that shouldn't be happening. So I went and saw a neurologist and had an MRI (which stands for magnetic resonance imaging—a way to take pictures of the inside of the body). Something showed up in those pictures.

At five years old, I was diagnosed with a brain stem glioma—a tumor on the brain stem.

Imagine a flower. The stem of the flower between the petals and the roots is like the brain stem. The most essential things pass through that flower stem—the sunlight collected by the petals, and the nutrients from the roots in the soil. Without the stem, the plant cannot survive. The brain stem is as vital to us as the flower's stem is vital to the flower. The brain stem is in the very center of the brain, at the base of the skull where the spinal cord connects with the brain.

In the brain stem, breathing, seeing, hearing, walking, talking, and swallowing, among other vital functions, are controlled. The brain stem is one of the most, if not *the* most, important parts of our body.

Tumors, in general, are classified as either malignant or benign. Malignant tumors (which are cancerous) tend to be fast-growing tumors and pose a dangerous threat to the "host." Benign tumors, on the other hand, tend not to be cancerous. These usually do not seem to grow at all, or grow very slowly, as mine did. They are less dangerous and can be tolerated for a longer time than malignant tumors, which are capable of causing more damage. For diagnosis, tumors need to be tested to see whether they are malignant or benign. A biopsy requires a sample of the tissue which comprises the tumor. To extract a sample of a brain stem tumor would be a potential risk. It would be unfortunate if any other part of the brain were damaged in the process.

Because of its delicate location, my tumor was too dangerous to try to remove. Extracting a small sample of tissue to test through biopsy was also too risky—we were still not exactly sure what kind of tumor it was. Since then, the technology may have changed, but it was a great call not to biopsy the tumor so early on for me.

My tumor is categorized as a glioma, which means it popped up in the glial cells that surround nerve cells and are supposed to help them work properly. The two main types of childhood brain stem gliomas are focal gliomas and diffuse intrinsic pontine gliomas (DIPG). The focal brain stem glioma tumors typically show slow growth in one location of the brain stem and are focused in one spot. DIPG tumors, on the other hand, can aggressively grow to other parts of the brain. They are not a single mass like focal tumors. Looking at the research, one of them has a MUCH better prognosis than the other. Focal brain stem gliomas have a life expectancy of over five years (a good prognosis), while DIPGs have a less favorable outcome, a matter of months. But it's not just that simple. There are also different grades of glioma, the first grade being mild and slow-growing, and the fourth grade being aggressive and high cause for concern. I've read that 80% of brain stem gliomas are DIPG and generally do not fare well, while the other 20% are focal tumors.

At my early time of diagnosis, the doctors weren't certain what kind of tumor it was. There were a lot of unknowns. My parents didn't know what type of tumor I had either. They just knew there was something there that wasn't supposed to be there. We didn't know what it was, and didn't want to risk further injury just to know what kind of tumor it was. None of this registered for me. I was five. I was into Happy Meals and Nerf guns. But for my parents, the uncertainty must have been extremely difficult.

Whatever classification my tumor was, and is, it seems to be low-grade (meaning, slow-growing or non-growing). If it had been a more aggressive tumor, I wouldn't be here to tell you this story.

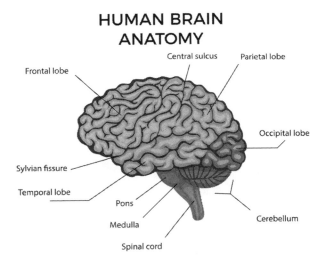

HUMAN BRAIN ANATOMY

Frontal lobe

Central sulcus

Parietal lobe

Occipital lobe

Sylvian fissure

Temporal lobe

Pons

Medulla

Spinal cord

Cerebellum

Many brain tumors are fast-growing. My slow-growing tumor has been considered benign (non-cancerous) due to the nature of its growth. However, it's always been considered high-risk due to its fragile position (at the ponsal-medullary junction of the brain stem). My official diagnosis is a brain stem glioma, but I've also seen it labeled a "benign neoplasm" in my medical records. (Image to the left is a diagram of the human brain. The brain stem connects the brain to the spinal cord, which carries nerves throughout our body. My tumor is where the medulla meets the pons.)

I've never known if I should think of my tumor as "cancer" or not. Lots of things I read indicate that a benign slow-growing tumor is not cancer, and other things I read say that all brain stem gliomas are considered "cancer" because of the delicate location they're in. Whenever the question "Are you a cancer survivor?" comes up, I never know what to say in response. I've experienced the neurological side effects, and have had radiation, but haven't experienced chemotherapy or the exact same struggles as (what I think of when I think of) cancer. But, in the end, the label doesn't really matter so much. What is in my head is what is in my head—no matter what it is. The focus hasn't been so much, "What is it?" as much as, "What are we going to do about it?"

The neurosurgeon discussed radiation therapy as a potential treatment, but when used on a child's brain stem, he explained, there is a significant risk of disturbing the natural distribution of hormones that glands (such as the pituitary gland) release into the body. We did not want to subject these glands to any radiation for fear of confusing my hormone distribution at so young an age. Any radioactive procedures would have to wait until after I had gone through puberty.

Some doctors told my parents my prognosis was poor. Their exact words to my mom were, "Mrs. Campbell, the prognosis for your son is not good."

Another doctor, who would later become my primary pediatric neurosurgeon for the next 25 years, did not give my parents the statistics. Instead, he gave them HOPE by providing examples of his patients with tumors, like mine, who were going to college and getting married. My mom later told me that was all she needed to hear to cling onto hope for me.

Survival Mode

Parents: Imagine your child is sick and you don't know if they will live or die. Or maybe you don't have to imagine because this is your reality. There's so much uncertainty about what will happen. And you have absolutely no control over the outcome.

For the first few months after I was diagnosed, my parents lived in so much fear that I wouldn't make it. My parents told me how helpless it made them feel—there was something, possibly growing, inside my brain, and they couldn't do anything about it. As they lived in fear and lacked joy, the owner of the daycare I went to pulled my mom aside and said to her:

"If Kyle survives this—great. But if he doesn't, you will have chosen how he lived his last few months on this Earth."

Those words penetrated my mom's heart, and my parents started living every day as if it was a wonderful day, grateful for each moment. If my time was going to be cut short, they would make sure it ended on a high note. My parents have maintained this attitude since that moment, and I'm confident that that positive mentality has been a tremendous influence for the benefit of our family.

I had MRI, after MRI, after MRI, to watch the tumor to see what it would do. I've probably had at least 40 MRIs, and I'm going to keep having them for the rest of my life. Whenever I'd go in to get my MRI checkup, the hospital staff would tell me how it was going to go, saying, "Okay, lie down here on this table, don't move, and halfway through, we're going to give you an injection."

After a few dozen times of hearing this, I'd say (or, at least in my head, I'd say), "Yeah, yeah—let's get this show on the road. I know what I'm doing here." (See image below: A magnetic resonance imaging machine uses a large magnet to take photos of organs inside our bodies.)

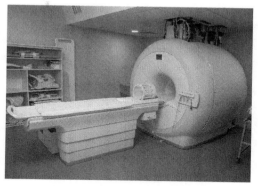

When I was younger, my mom would go in the MRI room with me to rub my feet as the gigantic machine took pictures of my brain. The MRIs would take about an hour. In the MRI machine, I'd either fall asleep or think about eating Round Table pizza. The cameras made all sorts of strange noises, and one of them sounded like a machine gun. Around that time, I was really into Sylvestor Stallone movies. I would imagine Sylvester Stallone as Rambo shooting his machine gun (you know, that part in *Rambo III* when Rambo does his snarling yell and shoots up the room at the end of the movie). Anyway, I digress.

My symptoms began to show up in elementary school. I was nauseous multiple times per week. I'd vomit multiple times per week (even in my classroom at school in front of my friends) and I remember being so embarrassed that I was doing that. I was dizzy—oh man, this was terrible. Everything would be spinning, and when I'd lie down, the spinning would get faster and faster. I was immobilized. I'd have to sit still and wait until the spinning went away. The dizziness would happen several times per week, as well. I spent lots of time getting to know the elementary school nurse's office. If I were too nauseous or dizzy at night when I was trying to sleep, I would signal to my mom in the room next to me by knocking on the wall if I needed help.

To this day I can vividly remember what it was like. I specifically remember being so dizzy and trying to walk to the school nurse's office, slowly dragging myself along the exterior hallway wall because I was so incredibly disoriented. I would have fallen had it not been for the wall to support me. I can still feel the scraping feeling of that brown stucco against my right shoulder as I recall the long walk from the playground to the office for help. Everything was spinning around me. (It's actually really hard for me to write this. It's scary to imagine myself back in that place.) Imagine yourself stuck on one of those swirly-twirly amusement park rides, except the ride speed has been switched to the fastest setting, and you could not get off the ride, even though you desperately wanted it to end. That's the best way I can describe it. I finally made it to the office for help—without falling over. I wouldn't wish this incredibly disorienting and helpless feeling on anyone, and I hope I never have to experience it quite like that ever again.

I was also a physically weak child. Reading back on my medical records from that time, I see the phrase "failure to thrive" mentioned in a few different places. For a few years in elementary school, the other kids called me "Skinny Bones." I didn't mind or take offense; I knew I was skinny. I remember my dad telling me a story about when he made me a chocolate milkshake with a teeny tiny vitamin to get some much-needed nutrients into my body. Always skeptical, I smelled the milkshake before taking a sip and exclaimed (much to my dad's chagrin), "This smells like the vitamins I hate!" as he gritted his teeth.

One day in fifth or sixth grade, our class was practicing averages. The teacher asked us our body weight, and wrote everyone's weight on the board. When it was my turn to say how much I weighed, the number I gave was about half as much as any of my peers. There was a brief moment of silence in the classroom as I could feel everyone wondering, "Really? He only weighs half as much as the average person here?" My metabolism was high because my heart rate was consistently increased (100 bpm would be my resting heart rate at times). Also, my food intake was low because, 1) I was a picky eater, and 2) I was stubborn. If something didn't look or smell quite right, I might not even taste it. I didn't want to eat what I didn't want to eat. (I like most foods now, but I still won't touch cottage cheese.)

My mom worried that my small size back then would lead to me being bullied at school. When she asked one of the yard-duty workers at my elementary school if I was being bullied, the answer was (so I am told) that I was actually *friends* with all of the playground bullies. They, in a way, looked out for me. I remember a time after lunch (maybe in the fourth grade) when we were all walking down the hallway. I pulled out a Twinkie my mom had put in my lunch for a dessert after my sandwich. One of the kids I was with grabbed the treat and said, "Thank you," as he started to open it, but another kid in the group I was with put the offending kid in a chokehold and said, "GIVE HIM BACK THE DANG TWINKIE!"

I wasn't trying to hang out with the big kids so I could be protected (I didn't know I needed it, anyway), I just thought these kids were cool, and I wanted to be cool, too. I guess it pays to be kind to people, especially if they're bigger than you and you're in the fourth grade.

As I got a little bit older, maybe around the time I was 13 years old, I started caring more about what my peers thought of me, and I wanted to hide those parts of myself I began to feel ashamed of. I remember a particular time I was at a friend's house. There were maybe five of us boys there all hanging out when it was decided that we would climb a fence in his backyard and go adventuring in the field behind his house.

Any ordinary boy at this age would be excited about that, right? Not me—my heart was beating faster, and I started to feel anxious as I followed the group into the backyard. I knew I had a tough time with balance, and I didn't want to appear to these other boys as if I was incapable or needed lots of help to climb a ladder over a fence. And even if I did make it over that fence okay, *I would have a difficult time keeping my balance and walking on the uneven ground, a challenge I had experienced often.* And then I'd have to climb back over the fence after exploring the area to get back into his backyard! I didn't want anyone to know my secret—that I struggled to do things kids my age should enjoy doing.

So what did I do as we got to the backyard fence and saw the ladder going to the top, which required balance to climb? I made the obvious choice and said the first thing that came to my pre-teen mind to get out of there: "I just remembered . . . I've got some stuff at home I've got to do. You all have fun!" And then I bailed.

My family loved the mountains, and I'd always spend time with them there. But as a kid, whenever I would go to a higher elevation I would need oxygen. I couldn't breathe as well. My oxygen-saturation level (I called it my "oxygenation") would be in the low 80s ("healthy" should be 95–100 or so). The effects of decreased oxygen saturation include fatigue, among other things. I would need to breathe pure oxygen through an oxygen tank we'd have to bring along. Without oxygen at the higher elevation, I'd get tired very easily and wouldn't be able to do much. I remember needing oxygen at our junior high winter camps, our annual family camping trip, and many other times. There is one story, in particular, that's no fun to remember.

My parents at that time had an annual ski trip to Mammoth Mountain, California, over Memorial Day weekend. We rented a cabin, and our good friends were at a place down the street from ours. One of those nights was my birthday, and we were all planning on celebrating at our friend's cabin they were renting for the weekend.

We didn't know yet about the seriousness of my altitude sickness, but we were about to find out. I had zero energy at our cabin. My heart was beating quickly the whole time ("like a rabbit," my dad says) and I vividly remember feeling exhausted the entire time we were up there. Everything was a chore—even just resting on the couch was exhausting. I spent my time up there watching movies with my brother and trying to rest so I could gain more energy, which seemed never to come.

I'm not exactly sure of the elevation we were at up there, probably around 10,000 feet. I remember trying to walk down the street to my birthday party, hand in hand with my dad. I started walking slower and slower down that street, energy draining and struggling more and more with every step to stay awake . . . until I fainted and was caught in my dad's arms.

I woke up later at our friend's cabin, and we tried to enjoy the night. Now, I look back, and I wonder, what was it like for my dad at that moment when I fainted due to lack of oxygen, to be standing there in the street with his child passed out in his arms? (We never went back on a Memorial Day weekend to Mammoth Mountain.)

As we drove down the mountain, my mom says I "perked right up," as we got into lower elevation. It was easier for me to breathe at lower elevations. Breathing was less of a struggle as my body could take in more oxygen to fuel my muscles. For the next few years, we'd take a tank of oxygen with us whenever we'd go into the mountains. Whenever I would start feeling exhausted from the elevation, I'd breathe in some oxygen, giving me a boost of much-needed energy. I remember the plasticy-smell from the tube I'd wear around my nose connected to the oxygen tank. I didn't use it all the time, but I sure was glad to have had it.

This is what life was like for me at that time—and not just for me, but for my family as well. This is something that we all went through. We went from Survival Mode to Coping Mode, figuring out how to live with my diagnosis.

"I'm Doing Okay, Mom, Aren't I?"

As a youngster, all of these symptoms were normal for me—the nausea, the dizziness, and the weakness. I experienced these so often that they became routine. At night, just before I'd go to sleep, I often wondered how sick I was going to feel the next day. I remember my mom consoling me once, perhaps when I had been dizzy or at a doctor's office, saying that she was sorry these things were happening to me. I don't remember this, but she says my response was, "Well, mom, somebody's got to be me. Might as well be me."

I had a GREAT time growing up. I am fortunate to have been born into such a loving family. I had fun with neighborhood friends, going to school, and being involved in various adventures with my brother (usually dressed up as pirates or ninjas).

It was also just a normal part of my narrative to have medical stuff going on. My parents and I visited my pediatric neurosurgeon's office a lot, so he could tell us what was showing up on my MRIs and keep watch on any growth in the tumor. We were there so much I remember the layout of the doctor's office waiting room. My favorite part was the reception desk, where we would check in for my appointment. A large yellow M&Ms guy sat on the desk. The plastic figurine was an M&M dispenser and would pour out a handful of the chocolate candies when you'd pull on his arm. (They're still my favorite candies, by the way—just ask my wife!)

In the appointments with my pediatric neurosurgeon, the doctor would go through a series of short checks with me. He would start with checking my eye movement from side to side and tapping on my joints to check my reflexes. He'd move on to check my strength, by having me grip his hands and squeeze, and then he'd gently push down on my shoulders while I would shrug them to check my shoulder strength. The hardest test he'd have me do is standing still with both eyes closed (balance became harder when I couldn't see). Other challenging tests were balancing on one foot with eyes open and walking a straight line—I could only make it a few steps before losing balance. Another test would be him moving his finger around and I'd have to touch my nose and then touch his finger (wherever it was in front of me). The strength tests I was always good at, but the balance and coordination tests were hard for me to do. The doctor would run through all these tests pretty quickly so he could keep a handle on how the tumor was affecting me.

My coordination, especially manual dexterity, was (and still is) poor. When I was a teenager and still figuring out what career I wanted to pursue, my parents connected me with a career counselor. Part of the process involved me completing a series of aptitude tests, to see what I was good at doing. When I did aptitude testing for finger dexterity (like for factory jobs), I didn't even place on the scale! It's really hard for me to finely manipulate objects with my hands, which makes it hard to tie fishing knots or to fix items around the house. I still do these things, it just takes longer. While my manual dexterity didn't even hit the charts on that aptitude test, my skills were super high in English and written and spoken communication. For all of us in life, we are naturally gifted in some areas, and not so much in other areas. It helps keep me humble knowing that I have a hard time with something that comes easily to somebody else. But, the opposite is also true—I have certain strengths that come easily to me that others do not have. I bet the same is true for you, too, having some things that are easy for you and some things that are hard for you. Our natural strengths are our gifts, and our natural weaknesses are opportunities to grow. We are all different, and uniquely crafted individuals.

At the pediatric neurosurgeon's office, the rectangular waiting room was long and narrow. The chairs around the perimeter of that room were always filled with other kids and their families, packed in like sardines while waiting to have our MRIs interpreted and read to us. It was normal to wait several hours for appointments there. I remember the other kids from that office, waiting to see the doctor to discuss their neurological or brain issues. Some of the kids you couldn't tell were sick, while with others it was much more apparent they had a lot going on. My mom recently told me a story I'd forgotten about a young boy in that office waiting room who just wanted to be well enough to play baseball. This young boy was in no physical condition to play baseball—he just wasn't well enough to do so at that time. Me, on the other hand, I could play baseball and do many things. (I was clumsy and uncoordinated, but I could still do them.) My mom tells me I looked at her then in that office and said, "I'm doing okay, Mom, aren't I?" Even then, I could see other kids were having difficulties, also, and some were more affected by their illness than I was. I hadn't quite learned much empathy yet at that young age. Still, in that environment, I started forming what would become the foundation of compassion for others.

The first time I internalized there was something different about me was in the sixth grade. Our class was walking single file, and my friend behind me asked, "Kyle, why don't you walk straight?" I replied that I didn't know; it was just how I walked. That got me thinking: it's not just that I didn't walk straight; I couldn't walk straight. I didn't have the balance to walk straight. Sometimes I'd stumble, not knowing why. It was just the way it was. When I matched this fact about myself to the observation that "normal" people walk in a straight line (rather than stumbling now and then or having an awkward gait), it finally clicked that my normal, the dizziness and sickness and fatigue, was actually not normal.

I had always had these characteristics of a sick kid, but I never understood that they were symptoms of anything. I always thought, *This is just the way it is,* and didn't connect it with what my parents and doctors said about my having a brain stem tumor. I started to understand something different was going on with me.

Radiating Hope

At this point, I was in junior high, with my brain stem tumor still slowly growing. As a brain tumor grows, it presses and pushes against nerves and blood vessels in the brain, which can increase symptoms or impairments in how we function. We speculated that the tumor was benign, because it was not posing an immediate danger, even after seven years. Because there was no aggressive growth, we did not choose to operate (if we could treat the tumor without surgery, that was the best case scenario). Instead, my doctor advised waiting until puberty (where damage to hormones would be minimized) and then having a round of radiation. Radiation is a less intense treatment than chemotherapy, but is still effective and serious.

The largest my tumor got was just over three centimeters in diameter (imagine a regular-sized grape in your brain stem). The brain stem is usually eight centimeters long in an adult. If my brain stem tumor was three centimeters, and the typical brain stem was eight centimeters long, then my tumor took up over a third of my brain stem. I'm sure that's not the medically proper way to say it, but that's how it makes sense to me. My tumor had gotten big enough: the timing was finally right for treatment.

When I was about 13 or 14, I moved up to Sacramento with my mom for six weeks to get external beam radiation therapy. (We had to leave my dad and brother at home so my dad could work and my brother could go to school.) We had some friends living close to where I was being treated, and they graciously opened their home to us. Imagine inviting two people to live in your house for a month and a half—no small thing to ask. We were very grateful for this. I remember I did not want to stay in a Ronald McDonald house, as I didn't want to be around other sick kids. Staying in our friends' home with their dogs and family dinners was such a blessing to us and helped normalize our situation. I have fond memories of playing *The Sims* on my laptop there, eating "bacos" for dinner, watching "Ant Kelly" battle the ant invasion, and all the kindness we experienced from those friends who became our family.

The waiting room of the radiation clinic at Sutter Oncology had all sorts of different people. Some patients were younger than me, and most were older than me. I specifically remember one older gentleman who was also having radiation there. He just wanted to make it six more months so that he could attend his son's wedding. Think about that. He just wanted to be alive for a little bit longer so he could attend his son's wedding. He was a nice, peaceful man, but you could tell by the look in his eye that there was some discomfort behind it, like he knew he was at the end of his life but was desperately trying to stretch his time out, to make it last just a little bit longer. (I don't know, by the way, if the man ever made it to his son's wedding. I hope he did, though.)

I saw these kinds of people and was exposed to these kinds of things as an eighth grader—not every 14-year-old's everyday experience. I didn't realize it at the time, but these experiences gave me a unique perspective on the fragility and preciousness of life. This perspective helped me enjoy the short moments we have while we are here on this Earth. The way I saw it, everyone has their difficult times in life, and I was having mine sooner rather than later. True, I didn't think this far ahead at the time, but I did understand why I had to be there and put up with it (at least to the extent that there was something wrong with me, and it had to be fixed). I knew that as long as I hung in there and stuck it out, it would be over soon, and I could get on with my life.

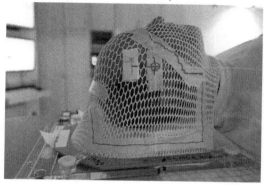

The stretch of radiation lasted for thirty days (five days per week, minus the weekends), a total of six weeks. At the introductory session, before we began radiation, I had a plastic mesh mask made that was perfectly molded to my face (an example is in the image to the left). During my daily radiation sessions, which lasted only 15 minutes, I would lie on my back on a metal table in a big room by myself. A gigantic 30,000-pound door would close to keep in the radiation when it was going on in the room. My head was bolted to this metal table by putting the mesh mask over my face and securing the mask to the table, so I could not move my head. During the radiation, a large machine (called a linear accelerator, pictured in the image below) rotated around my head to a specific position to precisely aim and deliver the high-energy radiation. And the laser beam was aiming for my brain tumor!

I received three small black dots as tattoos, the size of the end of a Sharpie, at different points on my head to help align myself with all the different parts of the machine in that room. During those

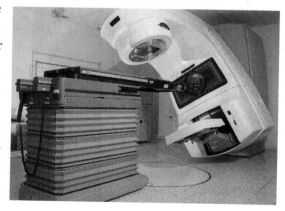

15 minutes of lasers shooting through my head, a red light in the middle of the room would flash to indicate the presence of radiation, accompanied by a loud buzzing sound to warn me that I'd better not move! After my appointments, when the technicians would help me off the table, I'd always leave with a slight waffle imprint on my face from how tightly that mask was fitted.

Every time I look in the mirror, even to this day, I still see those black tattoo dots on my face—one on my left ear, one at the top center of my forehead, and one on my right ear. They are not noticeable to the untrained eye, but for me, they serve as a reminder of having radiation. They remind me of lying on that cold, metal table and the delicacy required for that procedure. As an adult, I now look back at this procedure and I appreciate the gravity of the moment. There is no fear in these memories, but I can vividly recall the setting for such an important life event. At that age, I couldn't comprehend how this process was slowly saving my life.

The external beam radiation therapy was supposed to kill the tumor cells that were not supposed to be there in the first place. When I was alone in that room, lying on the table, I would wait until the red siren light started flashing and for the sound of the high-pitched whistle. It took more time to prepare for the radiation than the treatment lasted. The actual blast of radiation lasted only seconds. I was completely conscious throughout the ordeal. I had no sensation of pain during radiation, but I remember wondering how this was all working. This procedure would happen several times in a session, with my daily appointment only lasting around fifteen minutes.

When the radiation session was over for the day, we'd go back to our friends' house and wait for the next day's appointment. I was on independent study for school, and my mom helped around the house, so we had some things to keep us occupied. I also kept a daily journal on the laptop I was generously given before moving to start treatment. I posted my musings daily on a webpage I had, so friends and family could read about my experiences. Blogging, emailing, and instant messaging (does anyone remember AIM?) helped me feel somewhat connected to my friends back home during this time.

Back at home, my best friend would read my radiation blog every day in the junior high math class that I was supposed to be in with him. I'd have my school teachers telling my classmates what was going on with me, and I'd get emails from classmates that I didn't even know. The support from friends and family helped me through those times. When I returned during my eighth-grade year, I came back with a perfect rectangle of hair missing on top of my head (the "exit point of the lasers" where the radiation left my head). I thought it was neat that I was allowed to wear a hat at school due to my exposed scalp, while nobody else was allowed to wear hats on campus.

Mom and I made it the best experience we could. We had a great time staying with our friends in their house and visiting interesting places. We would also drive back home every weekend during my treatment to see my dad and brother. I listened a lot to albums by Jimi Hendrix on those road trips. (I don't think Mom was a huge fan of that, though.) There was a specific stop we would make, about halfway through the trip, where Mom and I would pull off the highway and get some In-N-Out burgers, fries, and milkshakes. That's also where Mom taught me how great it was to dip a burger into ketchup!

Waking up . . . but with Energy This Time

With my health the way it was as a kid, I had never really had lots of energy to be in good shape. I had done physical therapy with a family friend before when I was in junior high, to try to get some muscle where there was a lack of it. Being part of the medical community, a physical therapist has the education and professional expertise to come up with an exercise plan to alleviate or prevent pain, or for people with disabilities trying to maintain or restore muscle function. Physical therapy was very helpful with my balance when I was younger. *At the height of my frailness, Pilates-type workouts and strength-building regimens really helped me build muscle strength.*

A few months after the radiation was over, change in the tumor had not yet begun to show itself, but I did enter the "post-radiation slump." My body started reacting more to the treatment. The skin was sensitive on my head where the radiation had made its exit (where I lost my hair for a while). I was taking steroids to ease brain swelling. My appetite significantly increased as a side effect of the steroids, and I gained noticeable weight. I was always too exhausted to partake in much activity, so this period mainly consisted of me lying around and taking naps. I happened to make it home at the beginning of summer, so it was fortunate that I had the summer off from school. This constant fatigue lasted for a while but soon went away. I started feeling better and better.

As a result of the radiation treatment I received, along with all the powerful prayers coming from my home in Visalia, my brain stem tumor shrunk by about half—which, for me, has been monumental. Most of my symptoms were gone by the time I got to high school. I was no longer sick all the time, and I was no longer dizzy. I felt strong. I actually had the energy to want to get up out of my chair and do things without feeling exhausted. It was amazing how big of a difference in my body such a small change in the brain could make. I stopped getting dizzy, stopped having nausea, and stopped getting altitude sickness. I was now able to go back to the mountains without using an oxygen tank. No longer was I tired all the time, but I had the energy to go hiking, fishing, or do whatever I wanted to do (within reason). I just felt better overall, but my improvements would also continue, eventually turning me into a whole new person compared to who I was before (physically speaking).

My parents, wondering how they could help me with my physical state, got me connected with a personal trainer at our local gym. While physical therapy is all about restoring function, personal training is all about increasing strength and health after function has been restored. Personal trainers are fitness experts, and can describe proper form, techniques, and strategies for exercising in a gym. I only did physical therapy for a short while when I was younger, but I've had years of personal training.

The idea that I could gradually build up to something and eventually achieve it was put into me. It applied not only to the gym, but also to life. I'd start with baby steps, five-pound dumbbell curls, and the next thing I knew, I was beginning to feel physically strong. I noticed how much better I felt being stronger and how it made everyday tasks easier being more physically fit.

After not having had the energy to want to be fit, now I had the motivation, the know-how, and the ability to treat my body well and exercise. I'm never going to be one of those big bodybuilders, and when I go to the gym, there are plenty of people much stronger than me. However, knowing that I'm improving my physical self is good enough of a reward for me.

When I first started personal training, I would see my trainer at least once or twice every week. He would show me some exercises to do that would help me build strength and stamina, exercises that I could then later do on my own. The trainer and I worked a lot on core muscles, essential for balance and overall strength. The most important thing he taught me was motivation—how to motivate myself and use that motivation to persevere through hard work. This sense of motivation is still with me today and is readily applicable to many things. I used it to do long-distance running and hiking, and also things like earning college degrees, seeing a project or task through to the end, and even writing this book.

My poor balance is now the only thing I must battle with, and it makes simple activities (like walking, running, or hiking) that much harder. Using the motivation that I learned from personal training, I can persevere through these difficulties and do these activities any-way—even if it is easier to sit around at home.

I soon gained strength and got in shape, transforming myself from overweight and weak to average weight and strong. The dif-ference is amazing in how much better I felt. It became easier to breathe, easier to complete physical tasks, and I generally felt health-ier and more confident in myself.

Life becomes easier being healthy and fit. I don't mean that su-perficially or that people will like you more if you look trimmer (which is not true at all), but if you do not struggle with performing everyday tasks, you'll have more energy and will physically feel not so beat up at the end of the day. When you stay active, you'll have more energy to do what you want to do. You won't be so exhausted all of the time (I know because I've been on both sides of that spec-trum). I felt a greater sense of freedom in knowing that I could do more things that I wanted to do.

Growing up, I used to play a lot of paintball. My brother, dad, and lots of our friends would go up to a ranch in the foothills and wear an assortment of camouflage, split up into teams, and use the cover of hills, trees, and rocks to find out who would be the last team standing. (Usually, the team that had my dad on it would be the winning team, as he was more often than not the last one stand-ing. He's a natural-born hunter, that one—stealthy as can be!)

I remember I'd get so tired and couldn't do too much. All the other players would be running here, charging there, trying to get the upper hand in our paintball games, but it was always exhaust-ing to me to run anywhere. I'd usually find a good spot to shoot paintballs from a ways away to help my teammates. My dad got me a long barrel so I could sit back and shoot paintballs from a great distance—a paintball sniper barrel. This sniper barrel let me play without having to run around (thanks, Dad!). I was okay not being a main player, and was content to provide support to my teammates.

A couple of years after the radiation, the game was changed for me! The last time I played paintball, I experienced the unfamiliar feeling of having the energy to run to different positions to play the game. I wasn't a great paintball player, but I was even feeling bold enough to charge one of the best players we had been playing with all those years, a friend of my brother's. Of course, he got me out almost right away as I charged him. I knew I wasn't very good, but I didn't care. I felt great and physically strong for the first time in life that I can remember, and I wanted to use my new-found energy. (Really, I mean that—it was the first time I can remember feeling strong. And I was about 15 at that point.)

Things that were difficult to do before were now easier and more accessible for me to do. I finally had the energy I needed to want to do things. Before, doing something was always a chore for me, and I'd fatigue quickly. Now, I actually had the desire and energy to get out of my chair and do things. It's easier to appreciate something as simple as having strength and stamina when you went a while without it. I stopped worrying about whether or not I'd wake up feeling sick or dizzy the next morning (which used to happen there for a while). I started enjoying life for just how simple it was. I was grateful to be alive and experiencing whatever was around me. I was thankful that I could become a worry-free person.

I started becoming more of who I wanted to be.

Dream World: A Poem of Awakening

This poem was written at 14 years old, in October 2002—right after I had radiation and learned that it was really going to help me.

Dream World

I've been living in a dream world,
Most of my days.
It was a time of ignorance,
A time of play.

There were others in my dream,
But they were not the same.
This was my dream,
No one was to blame.

It was limited what I could do.
No one would know,
Nor have a clue.
I knew not who I was,
Nor why it was,
All until I heard that final buzz.

That buzz was the awakening,
It was my alarm.
It was my chance,
My lucky charm.

Now I am awake,
In the real world.

It would be exciting,
I would never be bored.

I enjoy everything now,
The people, the fun, the suspense.
All of this, I give my thanks,
To Jesus of Nazareth.

Challenges Persist

Even though a lot of my tumor has gone away, some of the nerves that were pressed and pushed against for so long are still impacted. The two main symptoms that I mainly struggle with to this day are my speech and my balance. My speech is different because half of my mouth doesn't work the way it should. The tumor slightly paralyzed the left side of my larynx (where the vocal cords are, at the bottom of the neck and throat). When we speak, air passes through our vocal cords, making them vibrate to produce sound. When not speaking, they should close completely to protect the trachea (air pipe) from food or saliva when we swallow. My vocal cords don't close all the way, so I'm more prone to coughing and have difficulty swallowing.

Swallowing can be challenging for me. It sounds simple, but it takes a lot of coordination in our throats (and coordination isn't really my thing). I remember as a kid coughing and trying to get my food down. My mom, concerned, watched me like a hawk when I would do that. I wanted to tell her every time, "I'm okay, Mom—no worries," but I couldn't speak when I was coughing. My signal that I was okay was to put my hands up in the air when I was coughing to let her know I wasn't choking and I'd be okay.

Also paralyzed was the left side of my pharynx (where the airway connects to the nose). Imagine a hole between your nasal passages and your mouth. When someone speaks, the gap is closed to give someone "the breath" to project their voice. When someone is not speaking, the hole is opened so they can breathe through their nose. This passageway in my throat was always open because the left side of that hole wasn't strong enough to close all the way. Because this passageway was always open, I never had the breath to speak. When I did speak, my voice would be soft (as I couldn't project my voice due to the loss of air through the nose), and my voice would sound very nasally. I couldn't regulate the airflow through my nose or mouth.

I remember as a kid trying to be friendly and talk to new people, and at times people would have no idea what I had said. They'd have to bring someone else in to listen or ask me multiple times to repeat myself. How many times can you listen to "What did you say?" before you get so frustrated you stop talking to new people? I already felt different enough; having people not be able to understand me when I spoke to them was isolating. I never knew who would understand me or who would return my greeting with an odd and blank head-tilting stare. I'm grateful that my friends who knew me could at least understand what I was saying.

I had speech therapy in public school from early elementary school until I was a sophomore in high school when I decided to stop going. Speech therapy seemed to not really be working for me after a point. I felt like no amount of practicing articulation could improve my hypernasality.

I heard my voice for the first time while lying in a reclining chair in a doctor's office. I was referred to an otolaryngologist (it's a mouthful to pronounce), who specialized in voice disorders, to see if anything could be done to improve the sound of my voice. The doctor had me "ahh-ing" with my mouth wide open as he looked at the back of my throat. As I was "ahh-ing" he took an instrument that looked like a tiny rubber hammer, and gently pressed against the soft palate in the back of the roof of my mouth—and that's when it happened.

By gently pressing on my soft palate, the doctor closed the gap that was supposed to be closed when talking (which my paralysis left always open). With that gap closed, I had the breath to speak. The voice that came out of my mouth when I "ahh-ed" I had never heard before—it was brand new. And at the same time, my voice felt and sounded so familiar, as if I had known it all along and had been searching for it all these years.

Hearing my true voice for the first time at around 17 years old (even though I was only making an "ahh" sound) was when it clicked that my voice could be understandable, audible, and clear. It was there all along, but my throat just didn't work the correct way to let my voice through. I starkly remember how much HOPE I had gained in that single moment, just by hearing myself make an "ahh" sound in a voice without any nasality to it—the sound my voice was supposed to be making all along. I knew, at that moment, that I'd do whatever I had to do to make that voice, my voice, permanent.

Getting My Voice

When I was 18, I had pharyngeal flap surgery to address this issue. A surgeon was able to make an incision on that left side of my throat and fold and move the tissue over a bit so that the passageway would close more. I remember waking up after the surgery. Imagine a sore throat, times a million—it was the worst pain I had ever experienced. It felt like someone had jammed a searing hot iron rod down my throat and pulled it back out. I immediately began to regret my decision to have surgery. I remember saying to my dad, "This was the worst decision I've ever made." However, it turned out to be one of the best decisions I've ever made. I was hooked up to a morphine drip in the hospital, which would give me a tiny bit of the painkiller whenever I pushed a button in my hospital bed. No matter how many times I pushed that morphine button to ease the pain (and I was pushing it a lot), I would only get a little dose every 15 minutes, and not sooner than that. (I remember "seeing" a giant talking teacup during this time, like the one from *Beauty and the Beast*, but the teacup was a lot bigger.) The pain eventually calmed down, and with the help of painkillers, I was able to leave the hospital and return home.

I had this surgery over Christmas break when I didn't have to go to school for a while and could spend my time resting. After the surgery, though, I couldn't eat solid foods for a while. While the whole family (cousins, grandmother, and family from out of town) was having dinner in the dining room, I was lying on the couch, munching on crushed ice cubes and feeling a little loopy on painkillers. (I remember my friend finding it so funny that I was loopy while on such heavy painkillers.) But as I soon discovered, the surgery and the ensuing pain were definitely worth it.

My reconstructive surgery was not about appearance, but rather about function. There was dysfunction in my throat and airway that needed to be corrected. Post-operation, I noticed that I was putting so much energy into talking really loud. This technique somewhat helped me communicate pre-op, but I didn't need to speak so loud now that I had had the corrective surgery. I could stop putting so much effort into my speech.

The sound of my voice significantly improved with added strength and no more hypernasality. It took me a while to get used to, and though it's still not perfect, it's noticeably a lot better than before. The number of people asking me to repeat myself drastically decreased, which reduced more of my self-inflicted stress and gave me more confidence in myself. Before, I wouldn't introduce myself to someone new and would be quiet around those people with whom I was unfamiliar. I was worried they would judge me before they knew me based on my speech problems, which has happened in the past. But mostly, it was all just in my head, stemming from a lack of self-confidence. Having a "regular" and stronger-sounding voice gave me more self-confidence, though it was not solely responsible for it. The decision to be self-confident was mine to make all along (I just didn't know it at the time).

It would have been so much more challenging to live my life without having this surgery. That simple change in the back of my throat has made my life so much easier. I can't express this enough. The number of times I was asked to repeat myself significantly decreased, making me feel an increased sense of belonging to the community around me. It was just such a relief knowing that I could communicate with people without having to strain my voice and without them having to strain their ears. Talk about a confidence booster.

After the surgery and recovery, I was given the breath to speak. Due to many years of speech therapists telling me to work on projecting my voice, and now that I no longer had to work so hard at that, I had to learn how to move my mouth when I spoke to best articulate what I was saying. I practiced. Whenever I'd talk to someone, I'd listen to myself and criticize myself. I would tell myself things like, *That 'R' or 'L' sound I just tried to make wasn't very clear—I'll try to say it differently next time.*

Sometimes it takes me a few seconds to coordinate the movements of my mouth and the sound coming out of it. I'll also start saying a word and repeat it if the sounds aren't clear, coming across as a slight stutter every now and then. I even had an app on my phone where I could practice my articulation. I learned to speak clearly and realized I needed a little more patience than I had. It's hard to diligently practice your speech. My mouth couldn't move fast enough to keep up with my thoughts, and due to the left side of my mouth drooping just a little bit, sometimes I had to focus a little more to get my words out clearly.

Since the surgery and lots of practice, I can (almost always) get through the day without someone giving me a blank look that says, "I didn't understand what you just tried to say," or asking me to repeat myself. Knowing that I am far more capable of communicating with people than before has improved my self-esteem. Thank God for surgeons! My speech is still something I'm working on, but I think it's been going pretty well.

I want to give a shout-out right now to all people with speech and communication disorders or barriers. I know it can be frustrating, and isolating even. I still have people who don't understand what I say. Don't let it get you down. Don't allow any negative thoughts about yourself to take root in your mind. Your voice is as important as anyone else's voice, and you belong. I hear you, and we hear you. Don't compare yourself to others. Spend time on what you can control—your own response to the situation.

Balance Barriers and Vision Difficulties

A major issue I still struggle with is balance—physical balance. The problem is that I don't have much. I don't have the balance to walk in a straight line, ride a two-wheeled bike, or do several other activities and tasks. Because half of my body is slightly out of whack, it throws off the whole thing. I need a wide base to stay on my feet, so driving a car isn't a problem because it has four wheels (and I plan on getting an awesome tricycle one day). My gait isn't straight, so it's challenging to run on a treadmill because I'm never quite sure where my feet will land, but I am sure that they *won't* always go where I want them to go!

When I walk or hike, I usually stumble and take extra steps to keep myself upright. The effort of taking those additional steps to keep my balance, paired with a naturally higher heart rate, means my body is exerting itself more to do the same hike as someone with a good sense of balance. I remember hiking in Sequoia National Park with a good friend of mine who wasn't stumbling all over the place like I was. I went on many hikes with him, and he asked me once, "Why don't you say much when we're hiking?" Ideally, we'd both be talking back and forth as we hiked. But, my body was working extra hard just to keep up and compensate for my lack of balance by taking those extra steps. It was too hard for me to talk because my body required extra effort to stay upright and keep up.

Even around the house, it's hard to stay balanced. I have to re-mind myself to slow down and focus more on my movements. I'm usually stabilizing myself against furniture or "throwing elbows" against walls to steady myself. Sometimes I'll start leaning one way and I can feel my balance going out of whack, so I'll do this thing where I spin around on my heel and catch myself before falling—I do this move quite a lot when I'm barefoot at home! Other times, I'll take multiple steps in a seemingly-random direction just to main-tain my balance (this move has been referred to as the "Kyle two-step"). My creative approach to not falling has been a fun challenge.

For a while, I was hiking a lot and it was always my goal not to lose my balance and fall. (I often fell anyways, so I got used to it and just got right back up.) I was on a hike one time with my dad and a family friend in the Mineral King wilderness area in California. We'd been hiking a pretty good distance, me with my trekking poles I always use. We were almost done with our hike for the day, and I felt pretty good about myself that I hadn't fallen even once on that whole hike! My dad was hiking behind me, and suddenly shouted "Black bear!" as he pointed to the hill across from the trail we were on. I quickly spun around to see the bear, and I lost my balance and fell. No! I had almost made it the whole way without a fall! Oh, well. Just get up and keep on going.

I'm likely to lose my balance, wherever I am, so I'm always trying to stay aware of my immediate surroundings so I'll have a plan for if and when I start to lose balance.

My balance can also get worse if I'm tired or sleepy. One day, some time ago, I was napping in a park before work. My alarm went off and reminded me it was time for my shift to start soon. I got up from the ground and stumbled a bit over the uneven grass, still groggy from resting. As I drove to work, I saw police lights flashing for me to pull over. I did, and found out I was suspected of driving drunk. As the two officers talked to me, I said, "I bet someone saw me stumble at the park and get in my car. Thinking I was drunk, they probably called you, right?" The officers indicated that yes, that was what happened. I don't blame anyone for thinking of safety or assuming I had been drinking. I'd be suspicious if I saw someone stumbling to a car and driving away. It just sucks that it has to be me. But, someone's got to be me . . . it might as well be me.

It was hard for me to do the breathalyzer test, as I already had issues with my throat and airways. I had to hold my nose with one hand so air wouldn't come through my nose as I blew on the breathalyzer. I understand that they had to have me do it to make it official.

The officers asked whether it was okay for me to drive with my brain stem tumor. I explained that balance wasn't an issue because a car has four points of contact with the ground. And then they left, and I walked into work. Not the typical start to your work shift.

Working out, staying in shape, and staying strong in my core helps me maintain my physical balance (for the most part). When I'm not regularly working out, I can actually feel my balance worsen. And when I am working out and strengthening my core muscles, I feel more sure footed. Being active helps me stay on my feet and improve my balance. I can vividly remember my neurosurgeon telling me, "Like a diabetic needs insulin, you need to be exercising." To maintain quality of life and not be stumbling all the time, I need to work out—whether I want to or not.

For so long, I was embarrassed at my lack of balance. I missed out on so many activities, making excuses for skipping events because I was ashamed to admit I lacked the balance to participate. I didn't want to try to participate if it meant I'd be stumbling all over in front of my friends. I felt like I had to say no to some of the things I wanted to say yes to. Now, I don't worry about that anymore. It's motivation for me to keep working out to maintain, or even improve, my balance and enjoy more of the things that this life has to offer. I've come a long way from that little boy, dizzy and stumbling along the wall to the school nurse's office.

Some challenges I've had for a very long time. I've adjusted and adapted to my balance being off. I have found ways of coping with it (slowing down, focusing on my movements, and leaning against objects), and methods for improving it (working out and staying active). My balance is also getting worse as I get older, but I'll remain flexible and adapt, when needed.

On the other hand, some challenges are new. Recently I've also acquired diplopia: double vision. It started when I was teaching in college and watched from the back of the room while students give their final presentations. I remember thinking, *Hmm, I see two of that student—that's weird.* To get rid of the problem, I'd just close an eye, and I would see correctly again. But after putting up with this for several years, I realized this was an issue that needed more attention than the brush-off I had been giving it.

When I finally went to the eye doctor, they diagnosed my double vision and set me up with prism glasses, which bend the light I'm taking in, so I only see one image (instead of two). I had never heard of prism glasses before and was pretty intrigued by them. If I don't have my glasses, I see two of everything—everywhere I look!

It's annoying. If I want to watch a movie, I need my glasses. If I'm driving, I need my glasses. I can make it without glasses for a short while if I concentrate, but it gets exhausting after a while. Even though I see double, my brain tells me where things are in relation to other things. Sometimes I

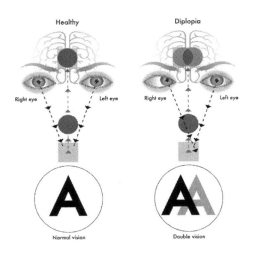

just put up with the double-vision if I don't feel like wearing glasses, mostly around my kids or someplace with not a lot going on. But if I don't wear them, I'll get headaches from concentrating too much after a while. (See the image for an example of diplopia, also known as double vision.)

My double vision seems to be getting worse, to the point where I still see double, even when I'm wearing my prism glasses. As I was reflecting on how I found an ENT who specializes in what I needed, I started to wonder if there was an eye doctor who would know more about my particular background with a brain tumor. I started researching, and found an eye doctor who specializes in neuro-ophthalmology (dealing with vision problems associated with conditions of the brain). This double vision thing is no fun, and a little disorienting. I wanted to do everything I could to help.

I didn't realize how important vision was until I had difficulty with it. The neuro-ophthalmologist was very knowledgeable and quick to understand my situation. When he saw "brain stem glioma" on my medical forms he said he zeroed in on that diagnosis right away. When I told him that I was diagnosed with the tumor at age 5, and had radiation at age 13, he quickly put together where my double vision was coming from. Eager for his answer, I waited through the explanation he was giving me. My double vision, he said, was most likely a result of the radiation I had when I was younger.

"Really?" I said, "even if it's now twenty years after radiation?"

Unwaveringly and confidently, he said, "Yes, it's definitely possible after that long."

I appreciated the perspective, and it made sense, but it was a lot to process. He further explained that the point of having the radiation treatment was to *damage* a *very specific* area in the brain, the area where my tumor was. Even with how precise and accurate radiation treatment is, it's still absolutely possible to have long-term effects from the exposure of that procedure to surrounding areas of the brain.

Twenty years earlier, radiation was instrumental in reducing my symptoms, improving my quality of living, and—who knows—maybe even saving my life. And now, after all that time, the "collateral damage" of that treatment was causing me to have double vision. It makes sense, when I think about it. My tumor causes *slight* paralysis on the left side of my body (visible in my facial expressions), so it makes sense that the eye muscles on one side might be weakened, also.

It's a lot to process, still, but I'd rather have had the treatment and be alive with some vision problems than to not have any vision due to not being alive at all! The uncertainty of what life will bring in the future can keep me guessing. If my vision could change after twenty years of having had radiation to the brain stem, what other changes might I experience? There are no guarantees in life. I need to stay flexible, faithful, and focused.

When challenges occur in life, we need to keep moving forward, keep adapting to our situations, stay proactive in our perspective, and maintain our focus on what's important. Challenges are opportunities for growth, and I want to make sure I don't step back when I am being called forward.

In Search of 'My Thing'

My family has always been active—not so much in the more traditional team sports, but more in outdoor activities. My family has always been big into snow skiing. I skied for a couple of years when I was younger, and it was a lot of fun. It was so thrilling having the wind whish past my face, turning and speeding down the hill.

I remember my last time on skis, around the age of 15. I had just gone up the chair lift and was on the top of the mountain. When I got off the chairlift, one of my skis slid out from under me, and I fell and hurt my leg. I'm not quite sure how it happened, but I knew that my injured leg wouldn't get me down the mountain—whether it was a pulled muscle, a sprain, or whatever it was. We had to call ski patrol, and they were able to get me down the mountain by laying me in a stretcher connected to the waist of the ski patroller.

Shortly after, I decided I did not feel confident on skis in the snow. My internal balance and coordination were thrown off. I just felt unsure of myself and not confident that I could stay upright. Balance is essential for skiing, and I was prone to losing my balance even if I was just standing still! I would still go to the mountain with my family, but I would choose to stay in the lodge and eat French fries instead of falling and hurting myself in the snow.

I was in search of "my thing"—something active that I could do. My family had skiing; I would find something else. My brother was on the wrestling team in high school, and I thought maybe I could do that. I went to one practice and realized that wasn't my thing, either. Not only did they work us hard to train, but I would be facing off with opponents who did not have balance problems. My doctor said I would be okay when down on the mat, but I knew

I wouldn't stand a chance when I was on my feet. I had to find a different thing.

I had to try something that did not have an opponent who'd outmatch me from the get-go. Around that time, my dad started cycling. I couldn't do that either—I didn't have (and still don't have) the balance to ride a two-wheeled bicycle. What would my thing be?

I asked myself, *What CAN I do?* I wanted to find my own thing, to help form my identity.

For college, I went to Cal Poly in San Luis Obispo, California. If anyone has been to San Luis Obispo, you'll know that it's full of outdoor trails. And right in my backyard at Poly Canyon was a great network of outdoor trails. I finally had my thing! I would start hiking and trail-running. It felt so great to just decide on something that would be my thing, that would be unique to me, and that I could physically do. I remember feeling glad I had finally found a way to be active and outdoors that was more reasonable for me to do—even before I had actually done any of it.

I remember feeling lonely so much of the time, like the people around me were doing things I couldn't. Now, I had something I could do, and it was only minutes away from where I lived. It was time to start my training!

I started running. At first, I could barely do a lap on the track (0.25 miles). Living down the street from our college track, I'd walk down every day and jog one lap, and then walk around the track for a few more laps. Over time, I gradually increased in distance as my endurance increased, and I slowly built up to doing two or three miles. When I was doing a reasonable distance, I began running on a dirt road that was uneven and went up and down rolling hills. There was a trail about a half-mile away from where I was living. I would run from my house, then along this trail, and at some point, would turn around to head back. As I ran more and more, I would gradually go farther and farther down the trail before I turned to start my return trip.

The trail was about eight miles long and sort of curved around into the shape of a crescent moon. I could technically go from my house to the beginning of the trail, complete the run, and then go back to my home in one full loop, but this was twice as far as I was used to running—I had to keep at it. I would be out there at least twice a week, seeing how far I could go once a week and using the other weekly runs to keep up my stamina. Every new week I'd increase my distance just a little bit until one day, I finished the whole loop, which came to about 9.35 miles. (I used a GPS watch to record distance, time, and heart rate.)

My finishing the route that day happened by chance, thanks to a giant cow blocking my return trail! She thought the middle of the trail was a great place to stand around that afternoon. Rather than try to coax and prod the cow out of the way, I just decided to keep going and see what I could do and how far I could go. That day, after months of running short sections of this dirt road, I completed the entire loop—out from my apartment, across the college campus, through the canyon, over and back down the hills, and back to my apartment. Exhausted, I returned to my house, stretched, drank a protein shake, showered, and fell asleep on my bed listening to the Lord of the Rings soundtrack.

When I first started hiking, I'd only make it half of a mile, then turn around. After doing this over and over, and gradually increasing my distance, I was hiking and trail running all over the place—I couldn't get enough! My body was finally able to do things like this. I did a lot of hiking and trail running in Montana de Oro, a state park on the California central coast. I did a 5k race, a few 10k races, and would hike all over the various hills and trails in San Luis Obispo. Later, I did some hikes in Sequoia National Park. I liked hiking by myself because I could go at my own pace without worrying about slowing somebody down. It felt like . . . *freedom*.

From being the kid who fainted before walking halfway down a street to being able to run on an uneven trail for nine miles and be active like this, I had come a long way—all because I had the idea that I could do it (and the medical intervention made a difference). I started by walking, taking baby steps, over and over and over, until I was running long distances. It took a long time, but the repetition, effort, and persistence produced results. This idea gave me the motivation that we all need to achieve great things, and all I had to do was reach out, accept it, and persevere.

The accomplishment might not look like what I had in mind when I started, but that doesn't matter. I wanted to run miles, and I started with walking a few laps around the track—but that's where I was. If we want to see things we've never seen, we have to do things we've never done. I had to start small (very small) for it to turn into something big. Failure wasn't a factor because I wasn't comparing myself to anyone else. My goal was to move forward. Taking small steps, even if I fell down on the way (which I did plenty of), I was still moving forward.

Adventures on Foot

The Scottish Highlands have always captured my imagination. Being of Scottish descent, a trip to Scotland was on my bucket list, especially after seeing how beautiful it is in the movie Braveheart. But, life was always getting in the way. As I graduated from college and started working, I started getting busy with everyday life. I kept putting this idea off as a dream apart. I started earning my own money, paying my own bills, and making my own grown-up decisions. There wasn't time to abandon everything and just leave the country—I had a life to build and get started.

While I was working in the group home I mentioned earlier, a coworker-turned-friend of mine was visiting town from Sacramento. It was winter break for him, a student of social work at California State University, Sacramento. We decided to catch up and go on a hike on the beautiful Central Coast of California, where there are plenty of trails to explore. He was telling me all about his adventures in South America. He had gone and climbed Machu Picchu to see the ancient Incan ruins in the mountains of Peru.

I was very interested in how he had just gone and left his life here for a trip like that, something I had never really considered. "There is no big letting-go process," he explained. "There is no getting your ducks all in a row. All there is to do is just go."

I knew that I wanted to go, and this was great timing for a journey like this. Being a young college graduate with no commitments or responsibilities, I was ready for the experience of a lifetime. I wanted my life to be an adventure and not just a steady for-sure job that may or may not have led to a career. I made up my mind that night—it was time to start living my life. That very night, I started planning my trip.

In July 2012, my cousin and I flew to Glasgow, Scotland. We embarked on a ten-day trip hiking the West Highland Way, starting from a small town called Milngavie (pronounced Mul-guy) and walking north through the Lowlands, skirting the entire eastern shore of Loch Lomond, then through the Highlands, and ending up in Fort William. We had a few days of traveling around the area after the walk. Still, our most memorable adventures for that trip happened on the Way. On that trip, we met people from all over the world, all walkers on the Way. There was a common mentality among us walkers, a shared affinity for adventure and new experiences. I remember feeling close to complete strangers just because we shared the craving for adventure and exploration.

This trek was tough for me. I had walking poles, which really helped compensate for my natural shortage of balance. Parts of the walk covered some pretty technical terrain (lots of rocks, tree roots, and things for me to trip on), which I consider my arch-nemesis. I needed lots of help from my trekking poles to stay upright. (Image was taken by my cousin while hiking a long ascent up a steep hill, with a valley behind me.)

Did I tell you how hard it was for me? It was hard. The most challenging part for me was not actually on the West Highland Way, it was a side detour we took. My cousin and I decided to hike Ben Lomond, a 3,000-foot climb and five-mile loop with lots of tricky terrain. I remember thinking that I couldn't do it on the steep hike up. Then I looked over at the trail and saw a young girl (maybe ten years old) going along with no problem, ponytail bouncing as she trotted along. I thought to myself, *If she can do it, I can do it, poor balance and all!* And make it we did—and the view was incredible. We have so many stories to share from that trip! There's the time we got stuck in the rain and shivered under a space blanket for an hour at the dock waiting for our ferry, the time we waded across a river to get to our bed and breakfast, and the time people thought we were missing and almost called search and rescue . . . but those are conversations for a different time.

It's true that I've done a lot of hiking and running, and have finished some neat accomplishments in that arena. However, I don't want to paint a picture other than what's true—I still have a hard time with balance and have had a hard time the whole way through. I've taken plenty of falls on hikes and have stumbled a lot while running (or even just walking, for that matter. I could even lose my balance just by standing still!). My feet don't always go where my brain wants them to go. I need to have my head down when hiking, focus on the trail and terrain, and concentrate on the placement of my feet. When I don't focus on where my feet go, I lose my balance. I'm no stranger to falling.

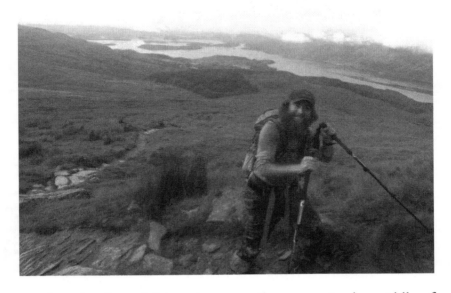

One day I was hiking along a trail way out in the middle of Montana de Oro, back in California. I felt (over) confident in my gait and coordination that day. I was thinking about how I always had to hike with my head down and looking at the ground. My friend and roommate, whom I did a lot of outdoor excursions with at that time, was able to look around and enjoy the beauty when he was hiking. I told myself, *Hey, I'm going to try that today. I'll get to look at the beautiful nature around me instead of just concentrating on the ground right in front of me.* I felt confident with that decision, thinking I'd enjoy my outing more if I were looking around.

As I was looking around while hiking, my foot landed on a rock, and the stone rolled under my foot, causing me to roll my left ankle. It was the worst sprain I've ever had. I have pictures of my ankle swollen up, black and blue, and not looking good. I chose not to pay attention to where I was putting my feet when I should have known better, and now I had to hobble back to my car! I winced with every step as pain shot through my ankle from any slight pressure on my foot. I was out pretty far and had at least a few miles to get back to my car to drive home.

I was wearing only my running shorts, and it was getting a little chilly as the sun was going down. I was going pretty slow as I shuffled down the dirt road, trying to beat the sunset to get to my car. At the same time, I could still see, and I remember passing a man on the road who was going the other way. As I painfully crept along, slowly progressing to help put the least pressure on my ankle, the passerby said, "Watch out for mountain lions . . . they start coming out at this time of the evening." *Great*, I thought. I was just trying to get back to my car to get the weight off my ankle, and now I had to keep an eye out for mountain lions! I should've known better and remembered to watch the ground in front of me when I was hiking. Finally after much pain and suspicion of shadows I thought might be lions, I got safely to my car!

Hiking and running are hard for me, but it's really fun, and I enjoy the challenge. Now in my thirties, it's harder than it was when I was in my twenties. I won't be able to do it forever, so I've got to enjoy it while I can.

Over the years, through trial and error of what helps and what doesn't help, I have learned to understand and manage my handful of conditions, or impairments. When those impairments are properly accounted for, I'm able to thrive. On one extreme end of the spectrum, I've been a sick little kid, dizzily stumbling my way down the hall to the school nurse's office. On the other extreme end of that spectrum, I've hiked 100 miles in ten days through rocky paths, up and down hills, and along dirt roads. One of my worst physical experiences, stumbling down that hallway, compared to my best physical accomplishment reaching the end of that trail in Scotland.

How did I accomplish this journey? It wasn't *just* through grit and perseverance—there was also a lot of patience and going at my own (slow) pace. Even baby steps in a direction is moving forward. Even if I set out to accomplish something and then I fail and fall on my face (which I literally have done multiple times), I'm still moving forward. When I fail at something, I learn a way it didn't work. I can adapt and use my learning to try something different next time. It's been a long slow journey through radiation, years of personal training, and experiencing other challenges to get me to where I was on top of that mountain—to get me to where I am today.

I am *convinced* that without experiencing all of my challenges and suffering, however hard they were at the time, I wouldn't have the resilient flexibility and adaptation, patience, empathy, and life perspective that I have now. I say with complete confidence: *It's been worth it.*

Embracing Disability and Disability Management

When I was growing up, I'd never heard of the word disability. The term itself wasn't talked about much that I can recall. It was when I studied rehabilitation counseling and learned about disability education that I realized I also have a disability. Or several of them. We learned about various "models of disability" (ways of understanding what disability is). A model that I am fully on board with is disability as a form of our identity. (I didn't actually learn about the identity model of disability in school, I learned about it while researching models of disability on my own).

We also learned about *visible disabilities* (those that we can see, and that have an external appearance) versus *invisible disabilities* (those others typically cannot see, the manifestation of which are internal or generally unseen by others). Sometimes, my disabilities are definitely visible, but most of the time, (I think) they are invisible (so I appear to be without disabilities). Most of the time, I don't know how I'll be perceived by others, but I'm ready to explain when asked. I've actually had a handful of people straight up ask me about my speech and what was going on with it. I used to be offended when asked about my speech, but now I'm honored by the honesty and curiosity of the question, so I take the time to explain about my brain stem tumor. Typically, there's a dichotomy between visible disabilities and invisible disabilities—a disability is either visible, or it's invisible. Brain tumors are neither and both, depending on the time of day, how tired we are, and other factors.

When I was younger, I thought I was the only person with this kind of tumor—I have never met anyone with this same kind of condition. But, I hear there's other people out there with childhood-turned-adult brain stem gliomas (and maybe they will even read this book, if they see it). I used to wonder where they were, and what their lives were like. And then I realized: Their lives are probably pretty typical in appearance, like mine. There's family, school, work, bills, sorting through junk mail, deciding what to have for dinner, calling their internet service provider every few years because they feel like they're paying too much for high-speed internet, and more mundane activities. There are also the extraordinary things, such as perspective and character, that these people live with.

Learning about disability education in college taught me that I had to *own* my physical disability. A lot of people don't understand the term disability and so it makes them uncomfortable. Especially in a culture that more or less *seems to* value ability and function, it is important to de-stigmatize and educate about disability. When I didn't know any better, I used to equate disability with less ability, and therefore, less value (in this ability-focused culture). I didn't want to admit that I had less value as a person due to limited ability.

Boy, was I wrong—about a few things. Everyone is different and has different levels of ability. The idea that ability has to do with value does not apply to people. A person has tremendous inherent value simply by being a person—no other condition needs to be added. Also, a person with a disability is not a totally disabled person. Persons with disabilities (like mine) still have lots of ability. (There is a debate about "person-first" language, such as *person with a disability*, and "identity-first" language, such as *disabled person*. I wanted to briefly acknowledge this conversation, but this, also, is a topic for a different time, with lots of "unpacking" to do).

It took me a long time to become comfortable with my disability and accept it. Now, I'm entirely comfortable and open with having my tumor. I *embrace* it as something that makes me unique, gives perspective to life, grows my resilience, and helps me connect with people. I definitely recommend anyone with a medical condition, especially other childhood-turned-adult brain tumor patients (if there are any others out there like me), to find out as much as you can about your brain tumor or health condition. The understanding and awareness of your condition, whatever condition it may be, is incredibly empowering.

I've included here an actual image of my brain from an MRI from February 2022, about 20 years post-radiation. I took this screenshot while screen sharing with my Stanford neurosurgeon. He explained that the tumor (circled and lighter in color than 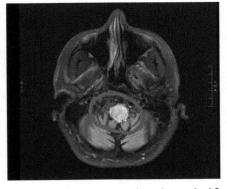 the rest of the image) had shrunk from its largest size by about half, but still remains and is still causing impairments by pushing against surrounding nerves and brain tissue.

As a child, I didn't question my brain stem tumor; it was just there and always had been (at least, I couldn't remember not having it). I was accustomed to doctors' appointments, and I didn't care much to learn about my condition back then. I was content to ignore it. As I became an adult, though, I started growing curious about the details of what I was diagnosed with and how it was impacting my life. This was not something I could ignore. Instead, I needed to actively manage and understand it.

Once I did my own research, talked to my own doctors, and read my previous medical reports, I felt so empowered! I could finally understand what was happening in my body and why I experienced what I was experiencing. I went from feeling ignorant and helpless about my medical status to feeling empowered, confident, and aware. Furthermore, I knew what areas of my health I needed to improve. Again, I recommend learning about your medical condition if you haven't done much of that yet.

As far as disability management goes, I also have the responsibility to take care of myself in ways that are unique to me. There are people in life who depend on me, and I need to be physically at my best to be the best for them. Have you ever thought of that? The better we take care of ourselves, the better we can take care of others.

I have already mentioned in this book the symptoms of the brain stem tumor I had as a child and now have as an adult, but I want to share about the ongoing *management* of my chronic symptoms and impairments that I live with every day: walking, speaking, and swallowing.

Walking: As I get older, my balance gets a little worse. While I don't usually fall, I do stumble quite often. I try to be very aware of my surroundings so I can throw elbows and balance with my hands against walls, lean my hips against a table, or use anything around me to assist in giving me more stability. If I'm ever walking next to you, I'm probably going to bump into you—repeatedly, without meaning to. My feet don't always go where I would like them to go.

To improve my walking and balance, I try to improve my

physical fitness by jogging or exercising. I recently got a new fitness tracker to help me stay on top of exercising (it does help remind me to be active). It's hard to stay committed, but I have to keep at it. Sometimes, I think about how I want to make sure I'm able to do things and be active with my family as my kids grow up. If I'm not extra-proactive with my health, it'll gradually decline.

Speaking: The clarity of my voice used to be poor. I remember the feeling when somebody would look at me with a quizzical look, trying to decipher what I had just said. It used to happen so often that I would grow frustrated and stop talking as much. I didn't want to get that look so often. I did have about 12 years of speech therapy in school, and I had that throat surgery to help me have more breath to speak with, but I needed more. I needed to do all I could to improve my speech.

I try to focus on my articulation and slow down with my pronunciation when talking, which helps quite a bit. I also recently went through voice therapy, to improve the strength of my throat muscles and diaphragm (to give me more breath to speak with and better sound when I do speak). I'd practice and learn about my speech and voice's clarity, efficiency, and physiology through my video appointments with Stanford ENT doctors. The most valuable things I learned from that experience are speaking with "Clearspeech" (which is deliberately over-articulating the sounds you are making with your mouth) and with a "forward" voice (which involves projecting the sounds of your voice out of your mouth, rather than keeping the sounds inside your mouth). I also practice vocal exercises, such as holding a note and raising and lowering my pitch, or an exercise where I purposefully over-articulate and slow down my speech. Since doing voice therapy, I've received unsolicited feedback that my voice has improved, and I'm more easily understood when speaking. So I guess the video therapy worked!

I still get the occasional look that means someone has trouble understanding what I just said. Sometimes I'll repeat myself to avoid the discomfort of someone trying to decipher my speech, or I'll switch the topic and play it off as if I said something else. I often repeat myself until I'm satisfied with the sound that comes out of my mouth. Sometimes it sounds and feels like I'm stuttering until I can focus and get the correct coordination with my mouth and throat.

Swallowing: I've had a sensitive gag reflex for a long time. As people, we cough when we choke on food to keep anything from going into our trachea (airway to the lungs). My throat often goes into overdrive and I cough to keep things out of the trachea, which is good, but it'll happen even when there's no danger of choking. It's called a laryngospasm. Things just tighten up to stop me from choking, and I can't breathe for a few seconds until my throat muscles relax. Sometimes, I'll have a laryngospasm when I'm neither eating nor drinking—it just seems to happen for no reason. It's no fun to be coughing and unable to speak, gasping for air. Sometimes when I'm coughing, or choking, or laryngospasming, I want to talk, but I can't, so I miss the opportunity to say something.

I cough a lot when eating, more than I used to when I was younger. For this reason, I try not to eat a lot around new people because I don't want to concern them with the impression that I'm choking a lot. When I do eat around other people, I have to deliberately bite, chew, and swallow with concentration. It takes me longer to eat, so I can try to coordinate my swallowing and minimize my laryngospasms.

The Stanford ENT clinic has been helpful during swallowing therapy. I've learned during a laryngospasm, I could sniff through my nose to trigger a reflex that opens up my larynx so I can breathe. (Go ahead, try sniffing right now—you might feel your throat and sinus muscles open up.) When I start having a laryngospasm and my throat tenses up, I can sniff repeatedly to help my airway stay open. (This has been an amazing thing for me to learn—thank you,

Stanford!) To help minimize provoking a laryngospasm while eating, I take smaller bites, chew more before trying to swallow, and have some liquid available to help wash it down if needed. I also practice a few exercises to strengthen my swallowing muscles. I'm still very likely going to cough when I'm eating, but at least I can minimize the severity a bit.

As a kid, I used to have lots of coughing fits. I would have to get up and leave the classroom for a few minutes so I could finish my coughing fit in the hall without disturbing the class too much. It was hard to walk when I was coughing and already struggling with balance, but I didn't want to be coughing uncontrollably in front of my friends. After radiation and throat surgery, my coughing was a lot better. But I still have a hard time with coughing and choking, to the point where my throat closes up and I can't breathe for a short time, and then it takes me a minute to recover. Sniffing doesn't always make it go away.

I'd been really struggling with my throat, and it seemed to have gotten worse since I was in my twenties. I remember when I realized that I needed to seek help for my constant coughing and choking. I was starting to feel helpless about my throat. The first time I found the online information for the Stanford ENT, I burst into tears. After feeling like there was nothing I could do to help my throat, now I found a doctor who specialized in exactly what I needed. I wasn't alone in my challenges like I thought I was. This was a huge revelation. I could use my resources to find my own doctors for various unique symptoms. I still have a hard time with it, but I know there are people to support me through it.

It's a similar situation with the neuro-opthamologist. A doctor who specialized in just what I needed, and they're in my hometown!

As I found more doctors specializing in effects from neurological issues, I started wondering about brain tumor support groups. They had never been mentioned to me when I was younger, so I grew up not knowing anyone else with a brain tumor. Even though mine is on the brain stem, there are a lot of similarities to other brain tumors people have. I've enjoyed reading the short accounts written by people with (or family of people with) brain tumors on the website for the National Brain Tumor Society, or NBTS. I see a lot of great survival stories on there, and people sharing about their difficult symptoms and their renewed perspectives on life. In particular, I totally agree with the perspective shared by someone who shared about "Finding joy in the mundane every-day things." That kind of joy can be found all over the place, and comes with *experiencing* the fragility of life.

Reading books and online descriptions of what people have faced with a brain tumor, I think my case has been mild as far as not having searing pain due to nerve damage, grand mal seizures, or headaches so intense I feel like my head will explode. I do have headaches sometimes, and multiple impairments in my activities of daily living (speech, swallowing, balance, walking, vision), but I'm so grateful for what I do have: life.

Disability management is a necessity for anyone experiencing disability or impairment (in terms of physical health, mental health, or both). Some conditions do not require much management, and some require a lot. My disability causes effects that I need to actively manage through things like doctor appointments, preventative exercises, and assistive devices (like glasses). To manage and strengthen these areas increases my overall wellbeing. It's a lot to work on, yes, but it's helpful and necessary.

A New Focus

My new self-confidence that came with my improved speech and balance (though neither was flawless) helped me relax and be content with myself. With the understanding of how my brain tumor impacted my body, I no longer blamed myself for my shortcomings. I knew what was happening now. I was not to blame for my health problems, just as I had no control over what color my eyes were or into what socio-economic background I was born. This was who I was, and I was no longer going to shy away from it. I used to be uncomfortable whenever anybody would mention me and brain tumors within five minutes of each other. Why worry about what we have no control over? It's just going to make us more stressed and anxious without the possibility of change. All we can do to change our lives for the better is to accept the situation and say, *Okay, here it is. Now what am I going to do about it? And if there's nothing to be done about it, where do I go from here?*

What helped me move on was realizing that I am in control of my response to situations and nothing else (such as other people or environmental factors). Realizing my lack of control allowed me to focus my energy on how I would improve myself. Letting go enabled me to do great things, like graduate college, get a job, get married, have kids, write a book, and, most importantly, be joyful.

Joy is a choice, a mental state, and a decision we make ourselves. It does not depend on circumstantial situations but on how we think about and interpret them. My circumstance is that I have a brain stem tumor, slight paralysis in my face, and am not very good at sports due to a lack of physical balance and coordination. As I get older, my symptoms (I don't know what to call them—my impairments?) will keep changing. What am I going to do about it? I will choose to be joyful. I genuinely want to enjoy life (it's going by quickly, you know), so I will choose to enjoy it.

Just as the Colorado River has shaped (and is still shaping) the Grand Canyon, life is an ever-flowing river of experience, pounding endlessly upon us and molding us into our unique selves. However, what makes us great is that we can interpret, learn from, and change our attitudes toward experiences and situations.

Throughout my life, I have had many seemingly unfortunate things happen. I burned my left hand at three and ended up in the hospital. I was diagnosed with a brain stem glioma at age five and ended up in the hospital. I had throat surgery when I was 18 and ended up in the hospital. Oh, and a few things (called "life") happened between being in the hospital. I've experienced multiple heartbreaks for multiple reasons (as I'm sure you have). My body needs more management to stay healthy as I get older (if you're over 30, you know what I mean). Not everything is smooth sailing. As I write this book, our family has been on a rollercoaster of events. Life happens, and it's hard. But we have to keep moving forward.

What am I going to do moving forward? I'm going to choose to enjoy every minute of life, hard or not. How am I going to do that, when life is hard and challenges and suffering come up? I'm going to choose to focus on the things I'm grateful for, and the things I can control. When the river pounds on me, I'm going to appreciate the beauty of the river. When I'm struggling to push a rock up a hill (Sisyphus, anyone?), I'm going to stop to appreciate the flowers along the way.

Life is good, and there is so much to appreciate in every single moment of it. Yes, it can be hard to shift our focus, but we *must* learn to appreciate it in the midst of the storm so we can move forward. The storms and rivers are coming, and we've got to be ready for when those moments arise.

I needed a solid foundation to help me move forward when the storms of life came crashing. I couldn't fight this battle on my own. It took a while to find, but I soon learned just how much more there is to this life than medical challenges and victories.

PART 2:
Faith and Philosophy

The Good News

The prognosis is often not good in patients with brain stem gliomas. My parents, who didn't know if their son would survive or not, found an incredible amount of support and community at our local church. They realized that they could not take this on by themselves. So they decided to put the issue in God's hands and found a church where they could get some help in doing this. They planted roots there, put their faith and my life in God's hands, and found some amazing people to connect with.

Every Sunday, I would attend church alongside them and my brother. Much of the time, I went to Sunday school to be with kids my age. I made some great friends and had some great times. In junior high and high school, I joined the youth group at our church. I was deeply enmeshed in the community, and we were all supportive of each other. For a 15-year-old, it was fun to hang out with other 15-year-olds to play pool and drink soda.

It was helpful to have people in our lives to bounce ideas off of who had similar value systems. I was going to some church-related event maybe two or three times per week by that time. It was great having friends that I knew would support me if I asked them.

I first learned about God from my parents and from attending church. There, we learned about how God sent His son, Jesus, to die for all people. God sent Jesus to die and pay the penalty for our sins so we could all have the chance to get to know God and grow closer to Him. Jesus willingly chose to die because He loved us so much; He wanted to give us the choice to live in freedom from sin and from enslavement to the ways of this world.

> *For God so loved the world that he gave his one and only Son, that whoever believes in him shall not perish but have eternal life.*
>
> *—John 3:16*

And not only did Jesus die for us, but He rose again after three days from death to life. If Jesus had just died as a martyr on the Cross, He would have been a prophet and a good teacher, nothing more. BUT, the difference is that Jesus was resurrected from death back to life.

> *Jesus said to her, "I am the resurrection and the life. The one who believes in me will live, even though they die, and whoever lives by believing in me will never die. Do you believe this?"*
>
> *—John 11:25–26*

This is the Gospel, meaning "good news": Everyone has an opportunity to know God. All we have to do is believe. And once we know God, we can know true Love and Hope.

If you declare with your mouth, "Jesus is Lord," and believe in your heart that God raised him from the dead, you will be saved.

—Romans 10:9

From Church to College

When I was about 16 and in the middle of my high school years, I experienced a split in the church I had grown up attending. Our family had tons of good friends at this church, like the people who had given me the laptop computer I used while undergoing radiation therapy. Our church community included people who had prayed, wept, and celebrated with our family. I'm not sure exactly what happened, but there was a leadership change. With the shift came differences of opinion on how to do things. Competing views seemed to disrupt many connections within the church. Some unfortunate things were happening, and I didn't understand why.

My church, where I had found stability for so long, was becoming an unstable environment. People were not compromising, understanding, loving, or even respecting each other—or so it *seemed* to me at the time. Some of the key leaders I knew in junior high and high school were leaving or moving around, and it was confusing to me why there would be so much change.

I decided that if these adults weren't going to act from a foundation of love, then maybe the church wasn't all it was cracked up to be. I still attended church, but for me it wasn't about God or learning about Jesus; it had become a social event where we would see friends once per week and sing some songs together. It stopped going deeper than that for me.

Through college, I became more focused on myself. I let loose a little (okay, maybe more than a little), but I never really did irresponsible things. I still had a good head on my shoulders from how I was raised. As part of the foundational beliefs I learned early on in church, I was taught to love and be kind to others. My family taught me to value others, and how to interact with people. (Mom and Dad, all those Sundays after church when you would talk to everyone about all kinds of things actually helped show me how to talk to people.)

I had to discover and explore the world for myself, and how I fit into it. Spiritually, in one of my writings, I referred to myself as a "theist" (one who believes in God). I didn't know there was anything else to add to that.

I had no idea what I was missing.

Journeys Through Philosophy

This section might be confusing for some and exciting for others. I write this for you to learn where I put my trust—and, ultimately, my Faith—and why.

When I was 18, I moved to San Luis Obispo to study philosophy at Cal Poly. I loved what I was learning and got really into it. At first, I wondered why I had chosen philosophy and worried that I'd never find a job. However, once I took a writing class called "Argumentative Logic," philosophy started making a whole lot of sense to me. In philosophy, you investigate things, analyze claims, and talk about why things are the way they are. Learning philosophy is learning critical thinking.

Looking back, I would never have changed my major, because of what philosophy is and what it pursues: wisdom and insight. Remember when I mentioned how I love the wisdom and understanding people can gain and share from their stories? One way of putting it is that philosophy is the insight of a story without the personal account—and that's what drew me into philosophy. That's what keeps me interested in philosophy.

I got super into analysis, science, and logic—maybe a little too much. Anything that was not related to those three was a waste of my time. I considered anything else inefficient, and I wouldn't deal with those things. Those things included emotion and faith. If I couldn't see it or understand it logically, I'd quietly ignore it and push it aside.

However, belief in God still made logical sense to me, based on several philosophical arguments, so I still held on to that belief. The world we live in is so complex and ordered, there *has* to be a Designer and Creator. Laws of nature, the biology and adaptations of organisms, astronomy and the expanding universe, and (being a dad) how babies are created, grow, and are born—all of these things are so incredibly precise and delicate. One Latin phrase I remember is *Ex nihilo, nihil fit*: out of nothing, nothing comes. All these things didn't just create themselves by chance.

> *For since the creation of the world God's invisible qualities—his eternal power and divine nature—have been clearly seen, being understood from what has been made . . .*
>
> —*Romans 1:20*

For my senior project for my Bachelor's degree, I decided to write an extensive research paper on knowledge. What it means to have knowledge, what knowledge is, and how we acquire knowledge is what I sought to explore. I thought that knowledge was what I wanted. Knowledge would answer why I had been given a brain stem tumor. Knowledge was the key missing from my life that would give it all meaning. If I could think about it, analyze it, and properly apply logic to the scenario, I'd arrive at my answer for why I had a brain stem tumor.

Why did I put so much emphasis on logic? Because logic is perfect. It's like math: two plus two will *always* be four—it just has to be. Some might say logic is a framework for how our minds work. Logic won't ever be wrong.

Unless a mistake is made in *our* reasoning, and people make mistakes all the time. I certainly do. I love logic, and I spent so much of my time in logic because I knew it would give me a straight answer. But, I didn't realize that, being human, I was capable of making constant mistakes and assumptions based on formulating premises from how things appear to me via my senses and interpretations. Logic is a perfect system, but my logical processes would be flawed (not all of them, but some of them would be) due to the assumption of premises based on my senses (which are not always reliable).

Once I realized my logic was prone to error (after being filtered through my senses), I started to see logic as untrustworthy as a system for testing the senses. Logic can only be relied upon 100% of the time when using non-observable information. If I was going to corrupt the system when applying it to my sensations, I shouldn't be trying to use it to answer every complex question. I had to move a little away from logic and put some of my eggs in a different basket.

I loved knowledge because it was true; it was fact, rooted in logic. But here's the thing about knowledge: a lot of what we think we know, we don't know—we believe. Science is incredible (particularly physics) for teaching us about the world we live in. It's how we come to discover things about the universe. But I would argue a lot of what we observe, we believe. Take the scientific method for problem solving. We're testing different observations and causal interactions, and then applying them to hypotheses. We support or deny a theory of how something is or the way it works through applying our observations to laws of nature. I would argue a lot of this leads to supported belief, as opposed to factual knowledge. We cannot factor in every possible variable because we could never think of them all.

Truth is real and exists, but some of it is out of our reach. Have you ever heard someone say, "There is no truth," or, "Truth is relative to the individual"? Well, those are truth statements. When someone says something like that, they're saying, "It's true that there is no truth," or, "Truth depends on the person—except for this statement, which is always true." Truth is out there, and we can grasp perhaps a tiny piece of it, but a whole lot of truth is beyond our reach. Some things that we think we *know* to be true, we actually *believe* to be true.

After my realization that logic couldn't result in the knowledge I was looking for, the knowledge of why I had a brain stem tumor, I took a step back. Instead of searching for a way to find the knowledge I needed, I realized that certain knowledge was, in itself, beyond our reach—and always would be, no matter how much supporting evidence we collected.

I tried answering my questions with logic and knowledge, and I didn't find what I was looking for. Rather than throwing in the towel, giving up, exclaiming, "Nobody knows anything!" and always living in the moment, we can and should form *beliefs* and have faith in how the world works—and how we got here in the first place. Not only that, but we need to be *diligent* in evaluating our beliefs for validity.

Considering all this, so many things I thought I knew were actually things I believed. And if I could have belief in something as observable and tangible as what science or my senses tell me, I could certainly have belief in things which science and my senses cannot tell me. I started wondering about spirituality and where it fits into all of this. It never made sense for me to argue on behalf of Jesus or God's existence or impact on this world because my logical reasoning couldn't result in that knowledge. But what if I didn't have to argue for those? What if I'd been asking the wrong questions all along? When I understood that I could only make sense of things as they appeared to me, a whole new world of beliefs opened up to me.

One of my favorite people from the Old Testament in the Bible, King Solomon, also thought knowledge and wisdom would give him all the answers. His story in the Bible says he was extremely wise, and if you have read Proverbs, most of which he wrote, you may see why he got that reputation. However, in one of my favorite books, Ecclesiastes, which he (presumably) wrote as an older man at the end of his life, he admits that seeking wisdom all your life is folly. What one should be seeking is God. In fact, nothing else matters, he says over and over.

I was led to stop pursuing knowledge and facts because it was an endless activity. There's an infinite number of things to know, and I'm never going to know them all. Pursuing an endless activity that would always leave me coming up short would kill me. As King Solomon (or whoever wrote Ecclesiastes) would say, *this is meaningless!*

I needed my life to have meaning. I knew that it did because I had experienced so much, and I felt that my story was meaningful. It was not all going to be in vain. I was going to use all of it; I just didn't know how. If my brain tumor had been just a little bit different, I might not have had a fighting chance to begin with. My question turned from *Why me?* with a victim mentality, to *Why me?* with an attitude of appreciation for the opportunity. Why was I chosen to share this message? And how could I maximize this message for the benefit of society?

I sought meaning in a different direction and found it. Or, actually, it found me.

Why Me? A Poem of Questioning

This poem was written in September 2002, right after radiation when I started asking myself why I had a brain stem tumor.

Why Me

Why me, o Lord, why me?
Why this, rather than everything?
Why me, o Lord, why me?

Do you have a plan for me?
And a plan for everything?
Why me, o Lord, why me?

What will happen, o Lord?
What do You see?
Why me, o Lord, why me?

Is there a reason, o Lord?
Only I can be?
Why me, o Lord, why me?

Have I been born for thee?
Perhaps to fight in Your army?
Why me, o Lord, why me?

Who am I, o Lord?
To fight the enemy?
Why me, o Lord, why me?

When will I go to spend eternity with thee?
Why me, o Lord, why me?

Skepticism to Faith

A friend of mine in San Luis Obispo invited me to check out his church when I was attending college. After declining his invitation several times, I decided to join him once simply because he had asked so many times. I had memories of the political drama in the church back home and half expected to see it again in this new place. But when I got there, I saw something my adult eyes had never seen before. I saw joy. I saw the love of Jesus on these peoples' faces and felt it in their hearts and greetings. These people were awesome, with unwavering attitudes of joy. Upon speaking to them, I learned they had challenges, just like me. Still, their attitude of joyful devotion to the Lord despite personal challenges was what intrigued me. I wanted that kind of life.

You never know when God is going to show up. (Little did I know, He was always there.) I lived in a 900-square-foot studio by myself that year, and I remember sitting at my desk with a Bible spread out in front of me. I knew many of these Bible stories from Sunday school, and I had even memorized a few verses. But, the Bible had never spoken to me. It didn't make sense to me, and I could never get into it. Reading those words always felt like a chore. I didn't see myself in them.

Have you ever felt that way before about the Bible? I bet some of you have. (Maybe all of you have felt that way at some point, who knows?) I didn't feel like it was relevant to my life. I had heard great things about it—how it changed people's lives and gave them hope. I had heard that it was the "Living" word. At that time, those words sure didn't seem alive to me.

But I kept looking. Surely, all those people who said amazing things about the Bible must have gotten it from somewhere. If other people were so inspired by what was found in the Bible, there had to be something to it. As I was thumbing through the pages, searching for what felt like a needle in a haystack, I randomly landed on the book of Ecclesiastes. I thought to myself, *Ecclesiastes is an interesting name for a book*, and I started reading to see what it was about . . .

> *The words of the Teacher, son of David, king in Jerusalem: "Meaningless! Meaningless!" says the Teacher. "Utterly meaningless! Everything is meaningless." What do people gain from all their labors at which they toil under the sun?*

> *—Ecclesiastes 1:1–3*

Whoa! This guy is a *teacher*, and he's saying *everything is meaningless?!* Very interesting . . . I had to read on . . .

> *All streams flow into the sea, yet the sea is never full. To the place the streams come from, there they return again. All things are wearisome, more than one can say. The eye never has enough of seeing, nor the ear its fill of hearing. What has been will be again, what has been done will be done again; there is nothing new under the sun. Is there anything of which one can say, "Look! This is something new"? It was here already, long ago; it was here before our time. No one remembers the former generations, and even those yet to come will not be remembered by those who follow them.*

> *—Ecclesiastes 1:7–11*

I was floored! I thought, *I could have written this! These are my thoughts!* Enthusiasm was pouring over me. I couldn't read fast enough. It made sense! And not only did it make sense, I saw myself in the Word for the first time.

> *Then I applied myself to the understanding of wisdom,*
> *and also of madness and folly, but I learned that this,*
> *too, is a chasing after the wind. For with much wisdom*
> *comes much sorrow; the more knowledge, the more grief.*
>
> *—Ecclesiastes 1:17–18*

This is where the rubber met the road for me. I'd been pursuing knowledge and wisdom for so long. And now, reading these words, which I could have written myself, I read that pursuing knowledge and wisdom leads to *sorrow and grief*?! I had to read on . . . and I read until the end of the book of Ecclesiastes.

> *Now all has been heard;*
> *here is the conclusion of the matter:*
> *Fear God and keep his commandments,*
> *for this is the duty of all mankind.*
> *For God will bring every deed into judgment,*
> *including every hidden thing,*
> *whether it is good or evil.*
> *—Ecclesiastes 12:12–14*

I had goosebumps. Is this what it feels like when the Holy Spirit shows up? (Spoiler alert: yes.)

It was the philosopher and theologian Soren Kierkegaard who wrote, "When you read God's Word, you must constantly be saying to yourself, 'It is talking to me, and about me.'" Reading Ecclesiastes that day was the first time I truly felt the Bible talking to me, and about me.

I'd always had the "head knowledge" that God existed and the Bible was true. Now I also had the "heart knowledge" that only God and internal experience could reveal. The passion and conviction that flowed through me encouraged my decision.

I started regularly going to church, Bible studies, prayer mornings, worship nights, and discipleship classes. After about a year and a half, I pulled my head up to look around, and I noticed that my life had changed. Overall, I had more hope, joy, gratitude, and enthusiasm for life. It wasn't because I was working so hard to understand the mysteries of the universe like before; I actually *stopped* doing those things and *let go* of the endless pursuit of knowledge. My life had changed because I started living a life of devotion to Jesus Christ.

> *But seek first his kingdom and his righteousness, and all these things will be given to you as well.*
>
> —*Matthew 6:33*

When we spend our time seeking and pursuing God and His kingdom, everything else falls into place. There is definitely no promise that following God will solve all your problems, but it will help you prioritize what matters in this life. God loves His creation (us), and He will provide us what we need. Not always what we want or ask for, but what we need and when we need it.

Now that I've had a relationship with Jesus and have chosen to live for Him rather than myself, I have found the answer to the question I'd been asking. Why do I have this brain stem tumor? Why have I had to face so much struggle in my life?

God was breaking my heart, over and over again, until it stayed open. And when it opened, there was room for Jesus to come in and consume me.

By choosing to look past myself to see the Lord, I finally understood. King Solomon said nothing else mattered than seeking God. Now I could see that everything else was fading and temporary, but only God was stable, and life and truth were in Him. I pray every day that God would use my hands to do His deeds and my words to speak His truth.

At this time, I was on social media. I posted a link to a great sermon I found talking about these and similar ideas. Shortly after posting it, I got a call from that same friend who used to read my radiation website updates in our junior high math class. He watched that sermon I had posted on social media, and he was moved enough to call me. He told me on the phone, *"Kyle, your life hasn't been about you. All the things you've been through . . . I've been watching. Your life has been about me."*

Discovering My WHY

My life isn't about me, and it has never been. It's taken me a long time to realize that. This was all really about what God could teach through me, by using my story, to help other people. Romans 14:7 says we do not live to honor ourselves, but we live to glorify God. So the way I see it, I was living for God's sake.

This fascinating epiphany, this mind-blowing revelation that I experienced and that changed my life perspective, has never been some Divine secret that nobody else knows. It was sitting right in front of me, in plain sight, in a book I'd read before.

One of my favorite books in the Bible is John, a book about the life of Jesus. I was re-reading it one day and, all of a sudden, it was brand new. I saw something that I had never seen before. In verses

1 and 2 of Chapter 9, Jesus is with His disciples walking down the street. The disciples see a blind man, a man who has been blind for his entire life, and they ask Jesus why this man is blind. Was he blind because he was being punished for a sin he committed, or maybe for the sin of his parents? Back in those times, if someone was experiencing some sort of disability, such as blindness, it was assumed that the person was being punished for some kind of past sin.

There is a blind man, and he has a disability. He has an impairment, and the disciples see this blind man, and they ask Jesus, Why is he blind? Why did this happen? They look back toward the past, toward the cause of this situation. They want to know why this man has this visual disability and what went wrong. What happened? Why is he blind rather than seeing? Did he sin? Did his parents sin? What happened? Who is to blame? Many people at that time in the first century believed that a disability like blindness was caused by the parent's sin. Jesus countered that belief.

When we have something happen that we think is bad in our lives, we often focus on the negative of the situation. Why did this happen? Why me? We try to figure out what went wrong. We try to figure out the cause because we want to blame someone or something. We want to blame sin, or we want to blame a situation. Or maybe we even want to blame someone for something that went wrong (besides ourselves, of course). We want to look for a reason why. Why did something happen?

I could ask (and have asked) my own question that way: Why do I have a brain stem tumor and why have I suffered in this way? Am I being punished for some sin? Did I do something I shouldn't have done? And, if so, what did I do? The answer that Jesus gives the disciples in verse 3, and the answer to that question that Jesus has given to me, is astounding.

"Neither this man nor his parents sinned." The man has done nothing to deserve this punishment. The individual has nothing to do with it—*it's not even about him*. Instead, this happened **so the power of God could be displayed in his life for everyone else to see.** It's not about the person or anything they might have done, and it's not even about what situation they might be going through. It's about displaying the power of God. It's about moving forward in hope in the midst of a challenge, not looking back for the cause of the situation.

Jesus did as Jesus does and gave a different, unexpected answer. Jesus does not look back. He does not look for a cause to blame for every problem. He does not try to rationalize or give a logical answer for why something is the way it is, something that we might understand. Jesus doesn't do any of those things. And I think we as a culture do these things. Something is wrong, and I go into defense and self-preservation mode, so I don't appear to others as if I have ill intentions. I don't want to be misjudged. And I immediately think, Okay, why is it wrong? What happened? Where can I put the blame? How can we make sure this does not happen again?

Jesus does not look toward the past. Jesus looks forward to the future, the possibilities, and the opportunities that might come from this. Jesus is more concerned about *how the man's blindness will be used* (future-focused) than He is about *how his blindness came to be this way* (past-focused).

So about the man born blind, Jesus says this happened not because of anyone's sin, but this happened so that the *power of God* could be displayed in his life for others to see. This happened so that the kingdom of God might be made just a little bit more magnificent, that it might receive some glory. Jesus can talk about the opportunity to display God's power. He was looking forward to what this might bring to the kingdom of God.

When we immediately jump to what happened, and we jump to why, and we jump to blame, we're missing the boat, we're missing the point. We should start by asking, What am I going to do with this? What opportunities might come from this situation? How can I use this to bring God glory? How can I use this to help other people? How can I use this to bless those who might need blessing?

The long journey to understand myself had finally reached a destination. With my own disability, for a long time, I asked why. And I looked for a cause or something to blame, an answer that made logical sense to me. And that sort of questioning didn't lead me anywhere except back to where I started. Looking back wasn't going to give me the answer I wanted and craved. Instead of looking back, I needed to look forward and ask, What am I going to do with this present situation? And how am I going to use it to bless others? How am I going to use it to bring glory to God? How am I going to use my own disability and my perspective to impact people?

I'm no longer asking why or looking for anything to blame. Jesus says it doesn't matter what the cause of it all was. Focusing on the why for too long is missing the opportunity. The opportunity is this: What am I going to do with this in the future? What am I going to do moving forward? With the perspective I have been given and the experiences I have lived, how will I use them to benefit other people?

I have been suffering from this brain stem tumor so the power of God could be seen in my life by everyone else through me. It has absolutely nothing to do with me. It's all about Jesus and how He can use my situation to bring Him glory and honor. Wouldn't you expect a blind man, or a person with a disabling condition, to be sad and melancholy about having some crucial aspect of their senses, like vision, taken away? And how much more meaningful and powerful would that blind man's story be, now that he has been able to say he was blind and now sees?

Of the small number of people who get brain stem tumors, most of them do not survive very long. If my tumor had been just *slightly* different, in location, size, or nature, I wouldn't be here. Surely, the fact that I'm alive is a miracle. I didn't realize this at all when I was younger, although I honestly don't know if I would have been able to really grasp it then. As an adult, this makes me appreciate every moment of life so much more.

I may not be 100% physically healed, but I'm ALIVE and very appreciative for the healing I have received. Doesn't it mean something more now that I have experienced sickness when I speak about the healing power of God? Doesn't it mean something more now that I'm so joyful and live with such a positive outlook, when I have good reason to complain and gripe each and every day about how I'm limited in my abilities? When honoring someone else, despite having experienced significant struggle myself, doesn't it mean something more to that person? By choosing to deny myself (not focusing on myself), I am able to honor someone else. Through that act, I am able to glorify God.

Sometimes, we don't even need to mention Jesus with our words to be a witness to how great God is. One of the people I used to work with asked me one day out of the blue if I was a follower of Jesus. I had never spoken to her about the church or Jesus—she had no way of knowing my beliefs. She just saw how I acted and my attitude, no matter the situation.

People see what you do, everything you do. They don't always comment on it, but they see how you act. How we act can preach the gospel—the Good News that our hope does not lie in this broken world alone. We have nothing to fear from this world because Jesus poured His grace upon us and died for us, giving us freedom from fear in the confidence that God will never fail us. The fact is that when we are on His team, He calls us children. Nothing can ever change that.

One of my favorite sayings is: Preach the gospel at all times and, when necessary, use words. Actions speak louder than words, and I want my actions to reflect the grace of God toward others. I've received so much of it, not having deserved any of it, that I want to pass it on and pay it forward. Not to try to pay any of it back (which is impossible), but because I want to obey the God who has freed me from this world, the God who commands me to love others as if I am serving Him.

God's power has been displayed in my life for all to see. My mission is to believe in Jesus Christ as God and make Him known as He who saves and redeems. I've learned that it doesn't have to logically add up because my mind isn't big enough to "make sense of it all." I can rest because it's not my job to figure everything out—all I have to do is live my life with faith, hope, and love. With confidence, I can look *beyond belief* and know what God has in store for us: life, and life abundant.

Trading My Sorrows and Fixing My Eyes

I didn't always like the path I was on. I prayed a lot to be healed, 100% healed. God had partially healed me through radiation and surgery, but I still have these impairments I struggle with every day. I didn't understand why He hadn't answered my prayers yet.

When I was going to college, I attended a church that believed in and performed healings through Jesus' name. I was a little hesitant and leery of it; I had never seen it before then. I vividly recall when I saw someone physically healed with prayer on the spot, and it was remarkable to see. One of our friends was using crutches (he had hurt one of his knees and couldn't walk around). After a few minutes of praying over his knee in Jesus' name at our prayer group, our friend JUMPED up and was healed! Never having seen a healing like that, I was skeptical. I asked him later how his knee felt, and he told me it felt great.

When the audience at church one day was asked if they needed healing, I went forward. I didn't like not having balance, and I didn't like my garbled, awkward voice. If I could get those things healed, that'd be great.

> . . . *whatever you ask in my name the Father will give you.*
>
> —*John 15:16*

I looked at the end of this verse, and I thought, *Whatever I ask, you say? Great! Let's go!* I went forward for healing at several prayer meetings. I prayed on my own for my balance and speech to get better. I wanted to be healed!

But I wasn't healed. The radiation had shrunk my tumor and alleviated many of my symptoms. God had kept me alive and protected me all that time, but He wasn't answering my prayers this time to heal the rest of my symptoms. And I was praying in His name!

Why were my prayers not answered to get rid of the visible signs of my physical disability? I prayed in Jesus' name to get rid of them, and they were still here!

A similar thing happened to the Apostle Paul:

> *Therefore, in order to keep me from becoming conceited, I was given a thorn in my flesh, a messenger of Satan, to torment me. Three times I pleaded with the Lord to take it away from me. But he said to me, "My grace is sufficient for you, for My power is made perfect in weakness."*
>
> —*2 Corinthians 12:7–9*

Have you ever *pleaded* with God for something? It's a remarkable word. When I think of *pleading*, I imagine utter helplessness and despair. I didn't like my imbalance or speech deficiencies. I was ready to be rid of these weights—too long had I carried them. Too long had they been afflicting me so.

My brain stem tumor and my physical symptoms are a constant struggle for me. Just like this verse says, they keep me from "becoming conceited." They keep me humble, remembering that I have a fragile body and am not invincible (as I once thought I was). Furthermore, just like Paul in this verse, I can recall those moments when I pleaded with God, fervently asking him to take away these thorns. Each time I prayed or went forward to receive prayer, I could feel the voice of God telling me, *Kyle, my Grace is sufficient for you. You don't need me to take these away. You need my Grace, and that's all. I've already offered it to you. All you need to do is accept it.*

There was one specific time when I went forward to receive healing at my church. As somebody prayed over me for my tumor to be healed and my speech and balance to be restored to their natural state (something God *can* do, by the way), I vividly recall that it just didn't feel right. I felt God telling me at that moment, *Kyle, this is who I've made you to be. There's nothing wrong with you, but this brain stem tumor **adds** to who you are and is how I've **designed** you to be. I want you to use this as an opportunity. If it's healed, your struggle won't be visible anymore and the opportunity won't be there anymore.*

The thorn in my side is my brain stem tumor. Have you ever felt tormented by a thorn in your side? Have you ever *pleaded* with God to take it away, and then it was still there, and you didn't understand why? *His Grace is sufficient for you, and His power is made perfect in weakness.* Whether you, or I, understand it or not.

I want to quickly unpack what it means to say, "My power is made perfect in weakness." When we are weak, we are not in control of our situation. When we realize we are not in control, we realize how much help we need to make it through. In that moment when we turn to God and admit that we need help and that we are not in control, *that* is the moment God's power comes out because we have realized it's not all about us. That's the moment we begin to look beyond ourselves for help. Then, we can let go of control and God will move.

Oh, and remember that verse in John that says God will answer anything we pray for as long as we ask in His name, and then He'll give it to us? Let's take a look at the first part of that verse:

> *You did not choose me, but I chose you and appointed you so that you might go and bear fruit—fruit that will last—and so that whatever you ask in my name the Father will give you.*
>
> *—John 15:16*

God chose me to go and bear fruit. Yes, He will be faithful to answer my prayers, but my purpose is to go and bear fruit. He chose me for that. I was praying for complete healing of balance and speech, but is that going to bear more fruit than thriving with visible disabilities and using them to talk about the Grace of God? I think the latter will be more fruitful. More challenging and uncomfortable, and also more fruitful.

The Apostle Paul wrote in Philippians 1:29 that he had the privilege of suffering for Christ. Paul was in chains because he would preach the name of Jesus, and people didn't want to hear it, so they put him in jail. Instead of sulking, instead of being sad about being in jail, Paul did all he could in that situation. He told the prison guards about Jesus; he told everyone about Jesus—as much as he could. And people listened to him because he was in jail, and they assumed he would be miserable. I imagine those prison guards were surprised to see Paul carrying out his mission. You know how when you see or hear something unexpected, it gets your attention? That's what happened here. It was unexpected to see a prisoner preaching love and good news while incarcerated, so it grabbed attention. Paul's attitude and words at that time brought those prison guards to Christ. Paul even wrote letters to various people and churches about how he was overjoyed to be behind bars for Christ.

Paul was in chains for Christ. And so am I. Paul had the privilege of suffering for Christ. And so do I. All I have to do is continue to take my eyes off myself and direct them onto God (which is easier said than done).

I've learned so much in my life through the experiences I've had, and I'm going to experience and learn a lot more things before my time is done on this Earth. I used to live a life where it was all about me: *my* thoughts, *my* feelings, and *my* concerns. I was arrogant enough to think I knew better than anyone else (really, I did for a while, I'm embarrassed to admit).

There's a lyric I love by Keith Green in his song "Make My Life a Prayer to You":

"It's so hard to see when my eyes are on me."

I grew up. When you grow up, you see things differently. Life gives perspective, gives experiences, gives stories, and gives lessons. Through my experiences, I've learned that life is not long enough to worry about discovering the reasons behind the things that challenge us. The way I see it, if you sit and just stew on whatever ails you, you're going to miss out and not find the incredible joys that this life has to offer, that God has to offer. I didn't want to miss out. I wanted to be joyful. But more than that, I wanted my life to have purpose and significance. And, boy, did I find it.

I've grown up, and I've seen how to be fulfilled. I'm fulfilled because I put my faith and trust in Jesus, in His name, and He'll never stop caring for me or supporting me in this life. He is the One whom I can always depend on, no matter what, to provide my firm foundation. Have you heard the parable about building a house on the shifting sand versus building a house on a solid foundation? I've chosen to build mine on the solid foundation of Christ, where the winds and storms of life, the struggles, sufferings, inconsistencies, and injustices of this world can never alter that foundation. This is how joy is possible in every Earthly situation. No matter what's happening around us, the truth and promise and hope of Jesus are always there.

Treading Upon the Heights

I heard on the radio a quote that I loved: "Just because you have the right of way doesn't mean the other cars are going to stop." In other words, just because we expect something doesn't mean it's going to happen. We can prepare for life to go one way, and then it goes another way and we're left trying to figure out what happened. God gives us the ability to be flexible and adapt to new situations, knowing that He will always be there and we do not need to worry—He'll care for us in any circumstance.

Since I've embarked on this journey of faith, I've taken my eyes off of myself and can finally see clearly. Life didn't quite go down the path I thought it would, but it's okay because life doesn't need to go the way I thought it would. I can still enjoy the path I'm on, and that's what I'm doing.

Though things didn't work out exactly the way I wanted them to, though my vision and my balance are getting worse, though the radiation I had to save my life is starting to affect me in more ways, though there are hard times in life . . .

> *Though the fig tree does not bud*
> *and there are no grapes on the vines,*
> *though the olive crop fails*
> *and the fields produce no food,*
> *though there are no sheep in the pen*
> *and no cattle in the stalls,*

yet I will rejoice in the Lord,
I will be joyful in God my Savior.
The Sovereign Lord is my strength;
he makes my feet like the feet of a deer,
he enables me to tread on the heights.
—Habakkuk 3:17–19

God "makes my feet like the feet of a deer." Nobody who sees me walk would compare my feet to the feet of a deer. A deer is extremely balanced and graceful when moving, and can even have such precise foot steps that they can step in their own footprints. They can walk along rocky ledges and suddenly bound in different directions, without losing their footing. The contrast is great—my balance doesn't allow me to do those things. So how does God enable me to "tread upon the heights" like a deer? Through any and every situation, I can have confident HOPE and JOY by setting my sights and focusing my life on things beyond what I see in front of me.

I first had the tremendous joy of sharing this message as a guest preacher in my hometown, and then was blessed by the opportunity to share at several other churches in the Central Valley. God had called me to share this message, and it was amazing to follow that call for the first time. I remember on one of my hikes around that time, I stopped to take a break from walking and I started preaching to a lizard I saw on the trail. Perched on a log with his head cocked, he listened diligently (or was staring me down—one of the two) while I told him this great news. We can have resilience to adapt to any situation. And yet, while we think we are weak, God makes us strong by reminding us that even though we are powerless on our own accord, when we rely on Him for our lives, tremendous things can happen.

But God . . .

After sharing my testimony for the first time, I was then asked to give the sermon on an Easter Sunday at a church in a small town. I came across this section of Scripture that stuck out to me. I wanted to talk about the importance and significance of what God has done for us, but I wanted to talk about it in a way I hadn't heard before. When I read this passage in Ephesians, I was inspired:

> *Once you were dead because of your disobedience and your many sins. You used to live in sin, just like the rest of the world . . .*

> *—Ephesians 2:1–2*

When I was in college, I didn't really understand the concept of Sin. I didn't commit any of the "thou shalt nots" in the Ten Commandments, so I was good. I mean, I accidentally stole a tiny pack of gum when I was little, but I apologized for that way back then. Before God got ahold of me, a Christian friend asked me once about my Sin and if I was guilty of any. I told him, "No, not really . . . I don't think so." I wasn't a bad person. I didn't do any wrong to other people, so I didn't think I was guilty of any Sin.

But here's what I didn't realize: Sin doesn't just mean being unkind to other people. Sin also means distance from God. For me, it was independence from God. He was doing His thing, and I was doing my own thing. I was calling my own shots, living my own life, and deciding my own path. I knew right from wrong, I didn't need God to tell me those things. Sure, God created everything, and nothing is greater than God, but I could take it from there. I was capable of doing it all (life) on my own.

I heard a sermon about the meaning of the word Sin, and I thought it was interesting, so I researched it myself. There are different meanings and connotations based on the language and the context in which the word is used, but one interpretation was about how the word for Sin has to do with archery. In this context, a "sin" in archery is "missing the mark" and not hitting the bullseye. The point of an archery contest is to hit the bullseye, and when you miss the mark, you do not get it right—you "sin."

"Missing the mark" applies to life—and to my life. I wasn't doing bad things against anyone and wasn't sinning in that regard, BUT I *was* sinning as far as missing the mark. I wasn't getting it right. I didn't have the proper perspective. I thought I would be okay doing things on my own, and that's not how life goes. We need God, for so many reasons, in so many ways. We are utterly helpless on our own. I've tried doing things on my own before, and it has never worked out in the end.

So, I lived in Sin. I was an expert at missing the mark. So what could I do now?

> *But . . . God, who is rich in mercy, made us alive with Christ even when we were dead in transgressions—it is by grace you have been saved.*

> —*Ephesians 2:4–5*

The crux of Ephesians 2:1–10 is that we once were dead (completely lost in sin and the ways of the world, totally obsessed with ourselves and our independence from God). BUT GOD loved us so much He brought us back to life and gave us a second chance, even though we missed the mark on our first try.

I want to make an important note about the words "*But God.*" The word *but* indicates something that came before whatever will be said next. For example, "It was this way, *but* now it's that way." It also *negates* to a degree what comes before by indicating an alternative scenario that is how things are. Imagine: "I thought it was this way, *but* it turned out to be that way," is saying that, in reality, it's not this way, it's that way. For example, "This is a great book, *but* I've read better," is saying there are other books better than this one, and to some degree, it negates that this is a great book by saying there are greater books.

"We were once dead, *but* God made us alive" means before God saved us, we were hopelessly lost. Once God gets ahold of us, that's when we start living. It's unexpected, yes. It's loving and merciful, yes. It takes faith to believe, yes.

Realizing how God has made Himself available to us, through Jesus Christ, totally shifted my perspective and priorities. It's mind blowing that the God who made all things, big and small, would care about me and my life.

He also cares about you and your life, no matter what it looks like right now.

Losing My Story

As naturally self-interested people, we want life to be all about us, where we're the hero of the story. After years of hanging onto *my*self, *my* story, what was wrong with *me*, and that it wasn't fair for *me* to have a brain stem tumor, I had to let go of myself to focus on moving forward. I've heard it said: Stop trying to find yourself inside yourself. Instead, you've got to deny yourself to find yourself. One of our local church pastors once said: "If you want to gain your life, you must lose your story." Or, the Bible puts it this way:

> *Whoever tries to keep their life will lose it, and whoever loses their life will preserve it.*

> —*Luke 17:33*

It's not all about me, and it's not all about you. We can find freedom from self-absorption in Jesus.

But here's the thing: Sometimes I still *want* my story to be about me! God has told me it's not, and I know it's not, but my mind drifts back to thinking it is about me. It is a constant battle to take that light off ourselves and shine it back onto God and others. It's easy to get caught in the spiral of self.

But, if we live a daily lifestyle of devotion *beyond belief*, we are able to keep our priorities straight and stay on the right path. Do not allow external, situational, and temporary distractions to throw you off course. When those distractions come, we need to first recognize them as temptations trying to keep us from pursuing our purpose. Second, we can deny those distractions any real estate in our minds. It doesn't work to just say, Okay, I won't let those things into my head—if we think about not thinking about them, we're still thinking about them! Instead, we need to occupy our minds with the right things so there's no free space to let in distractions. We can choose to pursue God and prioritize what matters, what makes a difference.

When we begin to share our identity in Jesus, we experience joy in every circumstance—even the painful ones. Joy is not happiness. Happiness is a temporary emotion based on external factors that affect us (I would say). Joy is a *decision* we make to trust God over our own understanding of things. We take comfort that we don't have to worry about controlling situations because He's the one in control. The good times, we will enjoy. The hard times, He can use for our good.

. . . We share in His sufferings in order that we may also share in His glory.

—Romans 8:17

Before we get to the presence of God, we must experience suffering. Whatever it might look like, the suffering people go through is an essential part of our stories. Suffering, though painful, brings invaluable perspective. Think about an especially painful season for you in your life—looking back, did that experience enrich your life perspective somehow? I bet it did, however painful it was at that time. I'm sorry it hurts in the moment; I really am. I want you to know we can have the strength to endure suffering because we know this present life is not our home, but we have a glorious Hope in the Promise of Christ and an eternity with Him in which to look forward.

Not only that, but if you allow Him to, God will REDEEM your situation and bring something beautiful out of it. I've seen Him do it over and over again, in my life and in the lives of others around me. It helps in the midst of suffering to wonder, how is God going to use this moment? How will He redeem this situation to bring something beautiful out of what seems so yucky right now? It can be tremendously hard to see the "good" when something painful is happening, but God promises (Romans 8:28) to work it out for us—and He's a God of His Word.

It's easier to look past suffering when it no longer dominates life. Furthermore, there is no reason to fear suffering. I even prayed for more suffering once, to teach me more about life. Really, I did. Unlike other spiritual traditions that suggest suffering is optional and escapable, Christianity says suffering is *necessary* for transformation to take place. Without the experience of suffering, we cannot rise to complete joy and freedom in Christ.

> . . . *Suffering produces perseverance; perseverance,*
> *character; and character, hope. And hope does not put*
> *us to shame, because God's love has been poured out*

into our hearts through the Holy Spirit, who has been given to us.

—Romans 5:3–5

Suffering is a stepping stone to the incredible freedom found in Jesus. I'm sorry for whatever you might be going through, and I'm sorry for how suffering feels in the moment. I promise: It's temporary, and (if you allow it) God can use that suffering for beautiful things, of which you have no idea.

Trust in the Lord with all your heart and lean not on your own understanding; in all your ways submit to him, and he will make your paths straight.

—Proverbs 3:5–6

We do not always understand. Not only that, there are some things we are not meant to understand. Don't spend your life looking backward, asking, *Why me?* Or, *Why this?* Instead, focus forward and ask, *How will this affect me moving forward?* And, *What am I going to use this for?* It'll be a much more fulfilling use of your time.

This is not my message to you. This is God's message to you. He's the author of where this all comes from, and I'm the messenger. Many other people before me have also given this, or a similar message, in different (and more eloquent) ways. But I haven't shared this before, and it's important you hear it from me, too.

PART 3:
Development and Emotion

Learning to Feel

I learned how to embrace my medical history in the introductory class of my master's degree program. There was an assignment to do a "Personal Development Project" to present what was most significant to us and our life stories. Unable to think of anything else with a bigger impact on my life, I presented on my brain stem tumor. To research, present on, and publicly own my medical history for the first time (in front of a group of people who didn't know my background) was incredibly empowering. I felt more confident about myself and how I'd gotten here. I shared about how fragile life really was, how close I came to not being here, and about all the miracles God has done and continues doing in my life.

The following semester, I took a class to teach me how to be a counselor. This class was supposed to teach me how to feel things, listen to people, and be present with them. This was challenging because these were skills that I had not really developed before. Listening, I could do. But, feeling?

When I was working on my Bachelor's degree studying philosophy, I considered myself a borderline stoic. I thought emotion was a bad thing because emotion would only get in the way of a task or an accomplishment. I wanted to avoid emotion. I did not want it to hold me back.

I had spent most of my life internalizing my emotions, so it was a learning experience developing emotional sensitivity to others. But, this was something I had to learn. God had called me to this program so I could learn how to connect with people, and I was going to do my best to be obedient to that call.

I remember the specific day that I learned how to connect with people on a deeper level. After my counseling instructor noticed my empathy was lacking, I received the feedback that I needed to work a little more on what it meant to be a counselor. I went in on a Saturday and met with two counseling instructional assistants to practice counseling with them.

At first, I didn't get it. I was just doing my usual thing and being my normal un-emotional self. The exact moment when I was able to connect on an emotional level, I was practicing being the counselor to the instructional assistant. She knew all the stuff that I was supposed to be doing as far as counseling goes. She talked to me about actual events in her life that were going on, things that were really hard for her. Trying to connect and thinking I knew what she was experiencing, I started smiling and nodding as she spoke. I recognized the feeling of grief myself, and I knew we could share that in common.

I thought, *Okay, I know what to do as the counselor here.* I smiled and nodded, preparing to say, "I know what you mean." She looked at me with a very straight and assertive face as I smiled and nodded, at the height of her grief and frustration. To my surprise, she suddenly exclaimed, "Stop F***ING smiling at me!"

I was shocked! It stopped me dead in my tracks. I had never really encountered such raw emotional intensity. I thought I knew what to do, but clearly, I didn't. Smiling and nodding during the height of someone's frustration and grief didn't make them feel understood.

It made them feel invalidated, unheard, and disconnected. I had to push aside my own discomfort with her pain to keep myself from interrupting her narrative and experience at that moment.

It was so hard to see when my eyes were on me.

It was not okay for me to be smiling and nodding right then. I didn't know what she was feeling, even though I thought I did. I needed to check myself and stop thinking of my own logical solution to her feeling of grief, frustration, and helplessness. I needed to listen and allow her to feel and be present in her discomfort. It's okay, and sometimes the best thing for us, to allow ourselves to accept and experience our discomfort and pain.

I didn't just learn empathy for others. I needed to allow myself to feel, and here's the thing about emotions: we cannot argue with someone that they do not have a certain feeling. We cannot and should not invalidate someone's experience of something.

When someone is sad, we sometimes want to argue with them and say, "I'm trying to teach you that you shouldn't be sad. You have so much to be happy about!" And how does that work out? Not well, I would imagine. Believe me—I've tried this approach for years!

We should still encourage each other to be grateful and to move forward. But, we cannot argue each other out of a feeling because the emotion is being experienced, whether it makes sense to us or not. We cannot argue against someone's experience of any emotion, the same way we cannot argue that someone didn't see something that they believe they saw.

Emotions are intrinsically tied to our behavior, inner dialogue, and even memories. Think about any memory you have that means something to you, that stands out to you. I guarantee that those memories stick out to you because you have an emotional attachment to those memories. Maybe it was a really happy time in your life. Or maybe it was a really sad time in your life. Or maybe it was a really scary time in your life. We don't always remember the content of the conversations we had, but we do remember the feeling of the moment and the environment. We have such a connection to the emotional aspect of events because they stand out to us.

God revealed to me just how important emotions are in our daily communication, attitudes, and even identities. Emotion is everywhere, and emotion is central to who we are as people—not just as individuals, but also as a collective society. I learned how important emotions are, and not only to empathize with other people and their feelings but to accept and understand my own emotions. I had to allow myself to feel things and stop myself from avoiding emotion—to accept that I sometimes have unpleasant emotions. Everyone has unpleasant emotions sometimes, and we all have wonderful emotions at other times.

We need to connect with people and be honest about ourselves. We need to be willing and vulnerable enough to share emotions, to talk about feelings. And I don't just mean happy feelings. We need to be genuine about what we are experiencing in life. Emotions are not a weakness—being able to *own* our emotions is a real strength. We will all have highs and lows, ups and downs, facing all kinds of things in this life. And we will have certain emotions attached to those events because we are emotional beings. We need to accept that. I think this is central for personal development.

People want and need to feel validated and acknowledged. Let's use our sense of empathy to listen to each other and imagine the perspectives of others. And if you need to work on your ability to connect with others, you can get better at it with practice. What can be more important than honing the skills that we use every day? What could be more important than knowing who we are and how we fit into this world?

I've been teaching a college class on personal development for a while. And I always begin by telling students, "This class is all about connection." How we connect in this society has so much to do with our personal development. Before we can connect with other people, we need to connect with ourselves. It's essential to think about our own emotional states, values, experiences, stories, and identities. Once we do that, we can learn how to share those and connect with others.

Connection and Community

Into the Wild is a movie based on the real-life story of a young man who leaves his family and college education behind. He travels from community to community, intending to get to Alaska, just to enjoy being in *the wild*. He gets there, and he lives on his own for a while. It's a great story, and I really enjoyed it. I'd recommend you check it out.

I remember telling my mom about how much I loved this movie, and I loved the adventure of just picking up and going. When I recommended the film to my mom to watch, she told me she'd already seen it, but she didn't want to tell me about it. I asked why she didn't want me to know about the movie, and she said she didn't want me to see it because she didn't want me to do the same thing and leave the family and never see them again!

At the end of the story, the main character comes to the realization that *happiness is only real when shared.* We need community. We need people to laugh with, share meals with, experience life with, and even go through pain with. When going through a struggle, community helps an incredible amount. It can feel so lonely when we are going through something and do not tell anyone. There's a misperception that we need to be strong, independent, and persevere to get through our yucky moments by ourselves. We don't need to do it on our own or prove anything to anyone. When we have people around us to support us, we can do far more than we can alone.

When we open ourselves up to let people in and share what we are going through, we're reminded that we are not alone. We're reminded of community—we do not have to carry heavy loads by ourselves, struggling to move forward. Instead, we can invite other people to share the weight of the burden, making it easier for us to get through.

> *Carry each other's burdens, and in this way you will fulfill the law of Christ.*
>
> *—Galatians 6:2*

No one needs to fight a battle alone. In the book of Ecclesiastes, it says nothing is new. Every situation has happened before, and people have made it through. You, too, will make it through—but we have to let down our walls. We have to be willing to be vulnerable first and not wait for someone to notice that we are having trouble. When you open up to people about what is going on, others will let down their walls to join alongside you in solidarity.

When I was first diagnosed with a brain stem glioma, my parents had a tough time. I'm told there was lots of crying and fear that I might not survive. My parents never would have made it through without a community behind and alongside them. My mom and dad got the devastating news that their little boy would have a hard time, and they needed people to help them carry that load through life.

They found this community in the Church. It was their Bible study group that gifted me a computer during radiation to encourage me to write. It was that group that showed up. It was that group with whom my parents have been lifelong friends and with whom they have been meeting for as long as I can remember. That's the kind of community and connection that can transform your life for the better.

I've noticed I find more community in my life when I reach out for it. In church, we spent a lot of time with our youth group, and I was connected to people there and in school. During radiation, people were contacting me who I didn't even know. They went to my school, heard from my teachers that I was having radiation, and wanted to message me to say hello. I loved talking with people. It helped me feel normal.

But, I never really shared with anyone about my tumor. The one time I shared what I was going through with someone, they didn't know how to handle that information and didn't talk to me as much after that. This made me not want to tell anyone. Don't get me wrong, I had a great childhood, great family, friends, and memories, but I just didn't share with people about my medical stuff. Nobody who didn't already know, anyway.

I remember it was *in college* when I first shared something deep and personal. I shared it on Facebook because I didn't know where else to say it. I wrote about limitations and how I used to limit myself to things, not take risks, and how I was done with all that. I didn't want to restrict myself anymore. I have an excerpt of that post, written on September 30, 2008—the moment I realized I had to share my vulnerabilities with people to build community (I'll remove the expletives):

> I have considered myself ruled by my limitations for most of my life. Anything I thought was hard to do, I naturally accepted that I could not do it. Now I've realized after doing some of these things that I control my limitations. My limitations do not control me. Now, when I am on the verge of

sorrowful regret, I realize my mistake. What I said wasn't just true of physical things. It is true of all things. I control my limitations. If I do not want to be limited, I will not be. Those who risk no loss also take no gain . . . which may, in fact, be worse.

One of the responses I got from that post was from a friend I'd grown up with. I remember him encouraging me and offering to help support me. Even though I'd known him for a long time, I never shared about my inner self, so he never offered to be there for me. I had never made myself vulnerable by talking about a struggle, and when I did, that's when he reached out to help me carry the weight of my burden.

People don't know you need help unless you say something. And we all need help. Reach out! Be willing to be vulnerable. You have nothing to fear in asking for help. When you ask for help, you are asserting your personhood. When you let your walls down to allow yourself to be open, genuine, and vulnerable, other people will take that as a sign that talking with you is a "safe space" and they will be more willing to lower their walls as well. Even though your feeling of fear is totally valid, don't let it control you. Remember, limitations don't control you: you control yourself. And if you feel helpless and totally out of control, ask God for help. When you are weak, He makes you strong.

Moving Forward

Growing up, my mom always made everything into a lesson. I'm sure we got a new lesson every day, depending on our situation. The focus was always forward: How can we use this? What can we learn from this? Our local church pastor would put it this way: "So what? What difference does any of this make for us?" I will put it this way:

NOW WHAT? After sharing my story and my faith journey with you, I will now do my best to give the application of its lessons moving forward.

Each day we are alive, that is one less day we have to live here on Earth—one less day to build a legacy, to leave an impact. How do we spend our time? Does it align with our values? More importantly, does it align with God's values? When asked to give an account of our lives, what are we going to say?

We need to be mindful and intentional to surround ourselves with the right things and fill our minds with the right thoughts. When I hung out with the playground bullies in elementary school, my dad used to tell me, "An eagle will never learn to fly if he hangs out with turkeys." The environment we choose to put ourselves into has a massive effect on how we act, impacting how we think and influencing who we become.

> *Whatever is true, whatever is noble, whatever is right, whatever is pure, whatever is lovely, whatever is admirable—if anything is excellent or praiseworthy— think about such things.*
>
> *—Philippians 4:8*

Every time I go to bed at night, that's one less day I have to live my life. I don't have time to spend on things I don't value. I don't have time to fill my head all day with negative news and the dark deeds other people are doing. What I think about affects my attitude, and my attitude affects my character, and my character affects my life and spirit. For this reason, we need to be highly on guard with what we spend the day thinking about. What we think about will affect who we become. Who we are on the inside comes out and shows on the outside.

God has shown me through my journey with a brain stem tumor what really matters in life. It might be subjective to people what's important or not important to them, but, for me, God shows me *daily* what matters and what doesn't matter. Things that are temporary do not matter as much as things that are long lasting. Things that do not impact others do not matter as much as things that benefit others. This perspective of recognizing important from not important has been one of the major blessings of having a brain stem tumor.

Our days are numbered; only God knows how many we have left. But the point is that we need to be intentional with aligning our short lives with the priorities to which we cling. Are your actions and your time aligned with your priorities in life? And for those of us in the Kingdom (we call ourselves Christians), are your priorities in life aligned with what God values? Faith, Hope, and Love are when we see past ourselves to something beyond. These are the major things which I seek and strive for.

> *And now these three remain: faith, hope, and love. But the greatest of these is love.*
>
> *—1 Corinthians 13:4–13*

Faith: *Faith is the belief in the unseen and unverified.* Whether it's based on external evidence (from our senses of things outside of us) or internal evidence (from revelations that God has given us), we all have faith in various things. I've heard that God will never give us enough evidence to eliminate faith. At some point, we have to decide whether to believe something or not. Based on what God has revealed to me, I have faith (belief) that He has a purpose for my life and that *that purpose is not about me but how He can use me.*

I also have faith God will take care of my needs, and He'll empower me to adapt to the various scenarios life throws at me.

Hope: Hope is not wishful thinking that one day things will just randomly get better. I'm not talking merely about the power of positive thinking or an optimistic view of life. I agree that those things are essential—but hope goes beyond those things.

Hope is the DECISION to have confident trust in God—that He will make a way for us through the storms of life, no matter how messy they get. Hope is confidently believing that God will use the difficult situation you are presently facing for something good someday, somehow. Hope has the power to change lives—your life and my life. No matter how dark things may get, there is always a little light if hope is there with you. There is always a silver lining to every storm cloud. In a life without confidence in God, either I'm left running the show, or the people around me are. I know I don't have total control of life, and neither do the people around me. I'd rather not have either of us be left in charge. I refuse to live a hopeless life. How about you?

Love: *Love is the merciful or graceful connection between or among living beings.* Grace is when we give each other good things not deserved. Mercy is when we choose not to give punishment that is deserved. When someone gives me kindness and I am undeserving of it, they treat me with grace. When someone chooses to forgive me instead of holding a grudge for a wrong I committed, they treat me with mercy.

We give grace and mercy in different ways. Love can come in various forms (romantic love, or friendship love, or a parent's love for their child). We need to be kind (graceful) and forgiving (merciful) to others—this is our calling.

Love is the greatest of these three because faith and hope are things WE have for God. Love is what God has for us. He has given us both Mercy and Grace when He didn't have to do that. Isn't that great! No matter what you have done, who you are, or what you believe, God loves you very much, right now, just as you are. There's nothing you can do to make God love you more, no strings or conditions attached.

Now we have the opportunity to love God and love others.

PART 4:

Lessons and Application

Living *Beyond Belief*

One of the greatest questions we can ask ourselves is: How are we to live? Given our individual passions, privileges, and perspectives, how should we apply those to the choices we make in life? Through both trials and triumphs, I have learned (and God has shown me) different ways of life to live by—to prioritize specific actions over others. We do not have time to waste on things that do not matter to us. Life is too short and fragile for that. My faith-journey has been filtered through the lens of a brain stem tumor, and that very faith has made my life so much more vibrant. This wasn't and isn't a story from my past—it's a story of where I am, right now, and the struggles, challenges, and joys I am still living.

These 14 tips are from me and how I strive to live my own life: beyond belief and with conviction. (I don't live up to these rules for living 100% of the time, but when I am off-track I try to get back to these.) Some of them have to do with each other or are closely related. I'd like to pass them on. Use them or not—it's up to you! You can use this section as a two-week daily reading and reflection opportunity, or you can read through them all at once.

1. Be Generous, and Let Others Be Generous to You

A generous person will prosper; whoever refreshes others will be refreshed.

—*Proverbs 11:25*

Growing up, I loved helping my dad with the yard. I was in charge of helping mow the grass, while my dad and brother would edge and trim. There were some days (as a teenager) when I didn't really *want* to help with the yard, but I had lots of experience with yard work. Because of this background, I readily volunteered recently to help a friend with his yard work while he was temporarily unable. It only took a few hours to load up the mower, mow my friend's yard, and come back home. I had fun doing it, actually, as I enjoy yard work. To me, it wasn't a big deal. But, to my friend, this small act of generosity meant a lot.

One day after work, I was walking out to my car to drive home. I couldn't find my keys, and I looked through the window of my locked car and saw my keys sitting right there on the front seat. I got out my phone, preparing to call Roadside Assistance, when a coworker saw what was happening and offered to drive me home to get my spare car key and drive me back to my car at work. After initially refusing her offer, I remembered how great it felt to be generous to people, and I didn't want to deprive her of the opportunity to be generous (and it was a safe situation for this person to give me a ride). To my coworker, it wasn't a big deal. But, to me, this small act of generosity meant a lot.

The world is a better place when we give and share freely. When we give things away, we remember that we are not tied down by our money or possessions. We can break free from the mindtrap that says we are worth as much as our net value. Imagine, rather, the value that you are building into yourself, your community, and others when you are generous. Some things are worth more than their market value. How we choose to use our time and actions can speak volumes. Let's break free from accumulation-mindsets and remind ourselves that our possessions do not own us. Let's be generous while we have the chance.

On the flip side of that, let others be generous to you. If someone offers to buy you something or do a small generous act for you, let them. Give them the chance to be generous towards you. By refusing their act of generosity, we are taking away their opportunity to help someone with something. Whether we need it or not, consider taking others up on their offer if they offer to be generous towards you. It's a great way to connect with people and build community.

Here's the challenge, if you've never done it before: The next time you're in a drive-thru line, paying for your drink or meal, ask the cashier if you can pay for the order of the car behind you. It's a great way to do something for someone, even a small act of generosity, that the other person does not need to pay back. They might even "pay it forward" and pay for the order after them. By being generous, we can know that we are giving to others whom we don't even know.

And if you are not in a financial position to be generous with money, be generous with your time. Time is way more valuable than money. Money comes and goes, and there's always opportunities to earn (or lose) more of it. But time is limited. Once it's gone, it's gone.

Spend a little extra time with someone, whoever it might be. Let someone else know they are worth your most valuable resource—your time and attention.

2. Be Kind, Even When Kindness Is Not Returned to You

*So then, while we have opportunity, let us do good to
people, and especially to those who are of the household
of the faith.*

—Galatians 6:10

I had just finished giving a presentation at a work event when I had
someone tell me I was "so nice." Rather than "nice" (which I think
of as a little passive), I prefer the word *kind* (which is more active, in
my opinion). Kindness is actively showing grace towards someone
by treating them with the professionalism, respect, and attention
that any person should receive. It doesn't matter if you agree with a
belief they have or not. We need to treat others the way we would
like to be treated ourselves—no matter how they are treating us!

Be kind. Everyone is going through something, fighting a battle
that we may not see or know about. They don't need our sass. They
need our support. There's a song called "That's How You Change the
World" by the Newsboys. It's about how small acts of kindness have
a lasting impact on people. Do you remember any moments people
have treated you with kindness? Likewise, people remember when
you treat them with kindness.

Here's the challenge: Be kind to someone today you think
doesn't necessarily deserve your kindness. This could be while inter-
acting with someone you don't know, someone with a different belief system or worldview, or even someone you disagree with about
something. The hardest part about this is putting our egos into
check. If we're not careful, we might presume that someone doesn't
deserve our kindness based on their actions. Since when did we earn
the right to decide who deserves anything? Are we better than others for having a different set of beliefs? It's called The Golden Rule

because it applies to any and every situation: treat others as you want to be treated—with kindness.

3. Be Patient

. . . be patient, bearing with one another in love.

—*Ephesians 4:2*

Have you ever had to wait? In line to check out at the store, for your kids to listen, to grow up, for other opportunities to come along—we wait on things all the time. What is it like for you when you find yourself waiting?

I waited a lot at doctor appointments. When my parents and I waited at my neurosurgeon's office to read my MRI results, sometimes we'd wait up to three hours for our appointment. It was just part of the routine, we knew there'd be lots of waiting.

When we are forced to wait and do not want to wait, we might start feeling impatient. We start fidgeting, feeling frustrated, and our thoughts are moving a mile a minute. When I'm feeling impatient, I start thinking about things like:

- What else I could be doing right now
- How this waiting is inconveniencing me
- How I could go about my life once this waiting is over, or maybe even what I could do to fix this situation, so I don't have to wait so long

But here's the thing: When I think about those things, who am I prioritizing in life? *My* day, the inconvenience to *myself, my* life, *my* actions. When we're feeling impatient, we are prioritizing ourselves. Is that what we want to be doing all of the time?

Being patient is being comfortable with the waiting. When we are patient, our minds are relaxed, knowing that we do not need to hurry this moment along. Instead, we appreciate the moment for what it is, and not just as another task on our to-do list for us to cross off.

Patience is not just passively waiting for moments to pass; patience is *actively choosing* to avoid the temptation of hurrying a moment along to avoid an uncomfortable feeling. Patience is choosing to sit with that uncomfortable feeling, knowing that whatever is causing the impatient feelings is the right thing to do at that specific time. Next time you are stuck waiting, and you start to feel impatient, *stop* the train of thoughts about yourself and *start* thinking about others. When we wait *for the benefit of others*, it's easier to be patient.

Here's the challenge: When you're at a store and need to check out, get in the longest line. Will it take a teensy bit more time to check out? Yes. Will it present you with an excellent opportunity to practice your patience? Yes. Will it give someone else an opportunity to possibly check out before you? Yes. (I used to do this at Costco and definitely had the chance to learn some more patience!)

4. Be Grateful

> . . . *give thanks in all circumstances; for this is God's will for you in Christ Jesus.*
>
> —*1 Thessalonians 5:18*

"Appreciate" is one of my favorite words. Why, you may ask? Because it has four syllables, and it takes a long time to say—especially for someone with a speech impediment that has to deliberately take the time to articulate each syllable of every word to be understood by others. Try saying, "Thank you." Now try saying, "I appreciate you." Notice how much more coordination and motion goes into your mouth when you say the second phrase. Maybe not a big deal to you, but it certainly is to me. I say that because for me to say *appreciate*, I have to really mean it. And when I hear others say it to me, I know they mean it, too.

What do you appreciate in life? What are you grateful for? Not just what are you temporarily happy about having around, but what are you truly thankful for? When we spend time thinking of these things, we are not spending so much time caught up in our self-absorption. We hold back the never-ending quest for the (temporary) satisfaction of getting or acquiring the next thing we have our minds on. Instead, we reflect on the joys of various objects or circumstances in our lives and their impact on us.

My wife put up a sign in our house that says, "When you love what you've got—you've got everything you need." Let's love what we've got, and spend some time on what we appreciate in our lives. The next time someone does something for you, let them know that you "appreciate" it. Pause and take the time to say, "Thank you, I appreciate it." And start making "appreciate" part of your everyday vocabulary.

Here's the challenge: Every night before you go to bed, write down one thing you appreciate. It could be every night for a week, a month, or a year—it's up to you. Don't worry if you miss a day. Keep your list going—one thing you are grateful for each day. You can go back and look at your gratitude notes in the future.

5. Be Intentional

*Be very careful, then, how you live—not as unwise
but as wise, making the most of every opportunity,
because the days are evil. Therefore do not be foolish,
but understand what the Lord's will is.*

—Ephesians 5:15–17

Intentional is one of my other favorite words. When we are intentional, we are doing things on purpose. When I see a person wandering around and appearing like they're lost, I can either remain
passive and do what feels safe—to keep to myself and mind my
own business—or I can *make the choice to act* and offer to help the
person find what they are looking for. Being intentional is making
that deliberate choice to act, on purpose, for the reason of helping
someone or accomplishing a task. Whether it comes naturally or if
you have to force yourself to do something, we can be *intentional*
about our lives and our choices.

As I've said before, we only have a short amount of time to be
alive here in this world. We are responsible for using our time wisely
to make an impact and leave a legacy. We all have the same amount
of time—24 hours a day, 7 days a week—and we can choose to be
intentional about our time. Being intentional means living our lives
on purpose, not just reacting to whatever happens around us.

Being intentional also means that I will say "no" to some things
that may not matter as much, so I can allow myself to say "yes" to
the things that I want to prioritize. I also think of the word conviction—when we are convicted, we know what the right thing to do
is. When God convicts us to act a certain way or do something, we
strongly feel that it's the right thing to do, and we need to act on
that call. Have you ever felt convicted to do something? And maybe

you didn't do it, whatever it was, and then you felt remorse for not following that conviction? When God calls us to action, and we don't answer the call, we realize later that we missed the opportunity to do something good or make a difference. Don't miss the opportunity! We need to be *intentional* about following our convictions.

I could be doing a million other things right now! Spending more time with my kids and wife, whom I love dearly, or even binge watching Star Wars or Marvel movies or shows, but I am convicted to write this book and share my story. It is the right thing to do, and God has called me to do it. I have to say "no" to some things, like going home on my lunch breaks, so I could say "yes" to other things, like using my lunch breaks at work to write this book. We sacrifice some things so we can prioritize others.

Here's the challenge: Make a choice today to do something you don't really feel like doing but know is the right thing to do. Tell a friend or family member about your choice and why you made that choice.

6. Be Resilient

Finally, be strong in the Lord and in his mighty power.

—*Ephesians 6:10*

Okay, we'll make this my last favorite word. "Appreciate," "intentional," and "resilient" all have four syllables—any word with four syllables you don't just say on accident (I don't, anyway). You have to deliberately say them *on purpose*. And you have to be or do them on purpose.

Resilience is being able to bounce back in the face of adversity. Resilience is having the endurance to make it through hard times, perhaps through reframing your perspective on experiences.

Resilience is being able to adapt to new situations when things are difficult.

Lots of people are masters of resilience, having to remain flexible and adapt to new situations. I can tell you from experience that people with disabilities are often masters of resilience. We are constantly having to adapt to new situations or symptoms, often having to creatively think outside the box to accomplish a task through an alternate method than normal. Poor balance? Exercise, lean against furniture, take extra steps, use your elbows or hands against walls to keep your balance. Poor vision? See an eye doctor, and then keep trying different approaches to correct your vision. There are multiple paths in life, and one is not "better" than another—it's just an alternate route.

It's okay when things do not work out the way you had in mind. You cannot always control what happens in life. So the question becomes: What are you going to do now? You will need to stay *flexible*, you will need to stay *faithful*, and you will need to stay *focused* on what matters.

Here's the challenge: The next time you are frustrated that things are not going your way, stop, breathe, and tell yourself to *smile, and remain flexible.* Change is one of the only guarantees in life. Remember that you cannot control every situation, but you can influence your response to situations. So, how will you choose to respond?

7. Make People Feel Valued

> *Do nothing out of selfish ambition or vain conceit. Rather, in humility value others above yourselves, not looking to your own interests but each of you to the interests of the others.*
>
> *—Philippians 3:3–4*

When someone honors you, they are making a statement that they value you. This could be paying attention to you, acknowledging you, giving you a compliment, or treating you with respect. There are multiple ways for someone to "honor" you. They are meant to make you feel valued.

I had a student recently bring me a candy bar. No big thing, it's a candy bar. But it helped make my day. Simple unexpected acts of generosity like that can have a big impact. Someone taking the time to think of you and do something for you, no matter how small, helps you to feel valued.

Other people like that feeling, too. *To look to the interests of others* means to actively look past your own value and intentionally *call out* the value in others. This is essential for connecting with anyone, and I believe we are called to do this. Before getting straight to business or jumping to the task you have in mind, make it a point to acknowledge someone's value. *Make others feel valued* and see how your connections with people jump to a new level.

Here's the challenge: When you see people and have small talk or even just say hello or goodbye, let them know it's good to see them. For a moment, prioritize them over yourself, and take the time to say, "It's good to see you," and mean it. People can tell when we mean what we say, and they will appreciate the acknowledgment, no matter how small. Also, use their name when you're talking with them. It makes people feel acknowledged and valued when we use their names. And if you know them but can't remember their name, you can say, "I'm so sorry, I'm a little embarrassed, I can't remember your name . . . ?" and they'll remind you. Furthermore, they'll appreciate your honesty and vulnerability.

8. Find the Good, Always!

Finally, brothers and sisters, whatever is true, whatever is noble, whatever is right, whatever is pure, whatever is lovely, whatever is admirable—if anything is excellent or praiseworthy—think about such things.

—Philippians 4:8

What we think about becomes what we identify with. What we allow to occupy our heads can influence our daily outlook on life. Do you spend your time reading doom-and-gloom news and stories all the time? You might tend to think negative thoughts about the world. Do you allow yourself to watch and get sucked into real-life murder mysteries? You might tend to be suspicious of people.

On the other hand, do you try to find the good in different situations? You probably have a positive perspective on life. Do you fill your head with uplifting stories of faith, perseverance, and resilience? You probably have an attitude of joy and a stronger sense of hope in the world.

I was raised with my parents (especially my Dad) pointing out the good. All those years of them trying to find the good in things makes me now search for the good in things. I find the good in things because I look for the good in things. We often find what we are looking for. What are you looking for?

We need to be thinking about what we are thinking about. We need to be intentional about thinking about things that are important to us and avoiding what is not important to us. The world is absolutely full of information. If you have a question about *anything*, you can look it up on Google! We don't have time to waste on thoughts that are not aligned with who we want ourselves to become.

When we focus on trying to *find the good* in the world, we train our brains to become more hopeful and optimistic about various situations. We find what we are looking for. Look for the good, and you'll find it.

Here's the challenge: Keep track of your thoughts. Every 30 minutes (or hour) for one day, record some of the things you are thinking about. At the end of your day, review the list. Are your thoughts "excellent and praiseworthy," or do they need to be adjusted to represent who you want to become more closely?

9. Put Your Focus in Check

Let your eyes look straight ahead; fix your gaze directly before you.

—*Proverbs 4:25*

Our feelings follow our focus. What are we focused on? What do we think a lot about? What we choose to focus on, we begin to allow ourselves to become. I had to put my focus in check when I was constantly focusing on the stock market. My focus was finances, and my feelings started to get wrapped up in finances. In reality, I don't want finances to be a priority in life, so I had to switch my focus and delete the stock market apps from my phone. Or when I do an over-abundance of research on buying "the best" of something. If I'm researching too much, my focus will get warped, and I'll need to step back. It doesn't matter if I have "the best" of something— having "the best" of anything is not my focus in life. What matters is that my focus and my priorities in life are straight.

If you choose to watch movies with cussing, you're more likely to cuss (whether it's speaking or thinking). If you choose to talk about drinking alcohol, you're more likely to drink alcohol. *Our choices can desensitize our inhibitions.* We need to be careful about what choices we allow ourselves to make. Let's ask ourselves: Is this choice to fill my head with these ideas going to align with my values and what I want in my life?

The same goes with *distractions.* With notifications constantly buzzing, screens everywhere, news and media flashing around us—so many things are trying to get our attention these days. A distraction is any unexpected thing trying to pull you away from your focus.

What are you choosing to focus on in life? Do you think what you spend time focusing on might be affecting your perspective in other areas of your life? Or do distractions constantly get in the way of what you are trying to focus on?

Here's the challenge: Make a list of your values. Write down your priorities. Are your thoughts and actions grounded in your values and priorities? You might need to refocus on what's important in life. What are some actions you can do to help refocus? (For example, turning off notifications, or setting alarms or reminders to make time for what's important to you.)

10. Consider It Joy

> *Consider it pure joy, my brothers and sisters, whenever you face trials of many kinds, because you know that the testing of your faith produces perseverance. Let perseverance finish its work so that you may be mature and complete, not lacking anything.*

> *—James 1:2–4*

How am I going to consider it all joy when it hurts so much? Have you ever felt loss or defeat? The hardest loss I could think of would be the loss of a spouse—a best friend and life partner. I've never lost anyone super close to me in this life, but if I did, and when I do, it would be absurd to consider it joy. Right?

My late grandfather was a Presbyterian minister, among other things, for a long time after he returned from World War II. I never got to meet his wife, my grandmother (my mom's mom). She battled cancer for a long time. When she died, at the funeral, my grandfather gave the eulogy (being a minister and her husband). I can imagine a large somber room, pews filled on either side with the people who had known my grandmother (who I hear was as sweet as can be, never said a negative word about anyone, and had a particular enthusiasm for life). I imagine maybe a quiet room, waiting for my grandfather to arrive and give the eulogy for his dearly departed and loved wife.

As he opens the doors to walk in, he enthusiastically bounds down the aisle between the pews, tambourine in hand, grinning from ear to ear and proclaiming, "VICTORY! VICTORY! VICTORY!" He takes the loss of his wife and turns it into a celebration that she is no longer suffering in her Earthly body and is now home with Jesus.

Is this example of suffering being considered joy absurd? Grandpa Jim didn't think so.

Challenges, suffering, and trials, of all kinds, mature our faith. For this reason, we can consider them joy. Look for the good. Be open to new change. Know that if you allow it, God will use your trials for something someday.

Here's the challenge: Joy comes from where we put our Hope. I have chosen to put my hope in God's unchanging foundation. The challenge for you is to think about where you put your hope. Do you have any hope to begin with? And if not, where can you get started?

11. Speak Life

Do not let any unwholesome talk come out of your mouths, but only what is helpful for building others up according to their needs, that it may benefit those who listen.

—Ephesians 4:29

The power of our speech and the words that we use is immeasurable. Years of verbal abuse can mentally incapacitate someone, and cause a lifetime of anxiety. And at the same time, years of verbal encouragement can build someone up to the point of doing great things with confidence and assuredness. Two very different uses of our words can yield totally opposite results—and they both come from the same source! Our words and tone carry so much power. If Spiderman has taught me anything, it's this: With great power comes great responsibility.

Sarcasm is using over-exaggeration or irony to mock something. As a kid I thought sarcasm (the mocking kind) was funny. I was always very quick with my wit to say something I thought was funny and innocent. I remember when someone told me once, in response to a sarcastic comment I'd made, "Kyle, you're so mean!" Even though that person was smiling and possibly being sarcastic back to me, I didn't want to be a mean person. I didn't even want someone to *think* I was a mean person. If a comment I made might possibly be construed as mean, I didn't want to say it. This is when I learned how important our words are.

Don't get me wrong—I'm all about humor! I like to use my quick thinking to make lots of puns, dad jokes, and one liners. (I do still exaggerate for humor sometimes, but only with close friends in non-mocking ways.) In fact, one of my life goals is to use humor daily to encourage people to smile. But, what we think we are saying isn't always what someone hears us saying. For absolutely everything we say, we should be asking ourselves: Will these words bring life or death? Will they build someone up, or will they tear someone down? How might this person, who doesn't know me as well, interpret what I am saying? I still sometimes think of those sarcastic things to say, but if they do not build someone up or add to the conversation I try not to say it. Holding our words back is a challenge, but a necessary one.

Here's the challenge: Be careful with your words. Don't use sarcasm to mock. Sarcasm seems like it can be funny, but really, it's disingenuous, dishonest, and disrespectful. Fight the temptation to add a snarky comment into a conversation because you think someone might think it's funny and boost your approval rating. (Jesus has already approved of you, anyway.) Say what you mean and mean what you say, being careful to choose your words to make sure they do not tear others down. Rather, try to choose words that build people up. Speak life.

12. Freedom in Forgiveness

Bear with each other and forgive one another if any of you has a grievance against someone. Forgive as the Lord forgave you.

—*Colossians 3:13*

My brother and I were young kids, and my dad was going to drive us to elementary school one morning. Already running late, my dad was just about to start the car as he looked in the backseat and asked, "Did you boys brush your teeth?"

"Yep!" said my brother.

"Yep!" I said as well.

"Kyle didn't brush his teeth," my brother said, exposing my lie to my dad.

My dad looked at me and asked me, again, if I had brushed my teeth. I knew I was busted. I confessed everything! Then, my dad took me inside, waited as I brushed my teeth, and clearly explained that he didn't lie to me, and he didn't want me to lie to him. Somberly, I nodded my understanding and awaited my punishment. He then told me he forgave me, and explained that he was going to let it go and not hold my wrong action against me. Once I heard that, I was grinning from ear to ear—my wrong was forgiven!

I'm grateful my dad took the time to teach me about forgiveness that day, even if it meant we were a few extra minutes late to school.

Have you ever had someone do something wrong toward you? Perhaps someone was too quick to blame you for something that wasn't your fault, or maybe treated you in a way that they should not have. Are you still hanging onto a grudge, or that one time someone wronged you? Are you still feeling resentful toward that person for that thing they did?

To forgive means to stop feeling resentful toward someone for something. When we harbor a feeling against someone for something they did, we are the ones having to suffer with that memory. To forgive is to let go of judgment toward others. When we forgive others, we are the ones who are set free. You don't need to forget about a wrong, but you need to forgive and move on. Otherwise, you're trapping yourself.

We are only hurting ourselves by refusing to forgive. Forgiving does not mean telling someone it's okay to do what they did, or that the wrong is acceptable behavior. It's allowing yourself and the other person to move forward in freedom from your condemnation of their past actions.

God has forgiven us. We need to be quick to forgive others, as well. I've heard that forgiveness is the greatest act of faith. Step out in faith, and forgive. Don't spend your time with an unforgiving attitude. We don't have time in this life to resent each other.

Here's the challenge: Forgive that person you've been holding a grudge against. Be eager to forgive. Don't allow bitterness toward anyone to take root in your heart. Live with a forgiving attitude. Do not hold a wrong or a grudge against someone. You can either forgive that person in your heart and move on, or you can let the person know that you forgive them. And the next time someone does something wrong toward you and says they're sorry, actually say the words: "I forgive you." Saying those words is meaningful because we don't always talk about forgiveness, and it gives the other person an opportunity to move on.

13. Let Go of 'Control'

In their hearts humans plan their course, but the Lord establishes their steps.

—*Proverbs 16:9*

Have you ever worked really hard to make something happen? You worked on it for a long time, dotted the i's and crossed the t's, planned everything out, and had all your ducks in a row. And then it didn't happen, and something else happened instead. We can and should plan, work, and strive to make things happen, but we shouldn't be surprised when things don't work out the way we planned.

I've done that before. I've worked really hard to get a certain job, and then I didn't get it. Or I made every plan so I could accomplish a certain task, and then something unexpected came out of left field and totally side-tracked my plans. I can work really hard to plan my course in this life, but it's up to God to determine what actually happens. The feeling of influencing my path makes me think I'm in control of my destination, when, in reality, I have absolutely no control over my final destination. Influence, yes, but control, no.

One of the greatest things I've learned is how to let things go. I still work really hard to plan things out and line up what needs to be done, but I've learned (the hard way) to let go of the final outcome of events. Don't personally attach yourself to necessarily having to acheive a certain specific outcome. Your path might yield other unanticipated and unforeseen outcomes—outcomes that have value that you couldn't see before. I can influence my path, and absolutely should persevere to do so, but at the end of the day, I'm not in control of the final outcome. And I'm perfectly content not being in control. It's a relief, actually, to have the pressure off.

I can't control the outcome of events, but I *can* control my response in the moment to whatever outcome I'm facing. God's got this, and He's going to see it through. This is the takeaway: I do not at all control the outcome of events, but I can determine my perspective. Outcomes are dependent on external factors, but our perspective is dependent on us and our inner dialogues. No matter what situation you find yourself in, you can always influence your perspective and inner thoughts.

Here's the challenge: Think of a time you worked really hard to achieve a certain outcome, but then for whatever reason it didn't happen. Did you feel like you were in control, at the time? What was it like to adapt to a different outcome? Was there any unexpected value of that certain outcome? Share with someone you're comfortable talking with about what "being in control" means to you in your life. And how do you feel about possibly not being in control all the time?

14. Live with Compassion

For the entire law is fulfilled in keeping this one command: "Love your neighbor as yourself." If you bite and devour each other, watch out or you will be destroyed by each other.

—*Galatians 5:14–15*

Many of us have heard the Golden Rule, to treat others how we want to be treated. Did you know this is where it comes from, in the Bible? God calls us to love our neighbors as we love ourselves—to treat others the way we would want to be treated.

If you look up the definition of "compassion" you'll find several different meanings having to do with wanting to help people. I think of "com" and "passion," where "com" is like community and "passion" is a strong feeling, so "compassion" is community feeling, or feeling together. It's not just sharing the emotions of another individual, but it's driven by a desire to want to help people.

Working at a college and with so many people starting out in their careers, I hear tons and tons of people say they don't know exactly what they want to do in their career, but they know they want to help people. I remember saying the same thing, myself: "I want to help people, but I don't know how or what to do."

We can live with compassion *right now.* We don't need to wait to earn a degree or get started in a certain job, or for anything else to happen, before we can love on others and help them out. Compassion is acknowledging someone's need, identifying with their feeling of need, and then stepping up to meet that need. Let's love our neighbors as ourselves and treat them like we would want to be treated—with patience and compassion.

Here's the challenge: Find someone in need of something, imagine what it would be like for that person to be in need, and then find a way to address that need. It could be an old friend who needs some encouragement, or a person feeling lonely who needs your company. Maybe it's an elderly person needing help with some chores, a family member needing your forgiveness for something, or a hungry person on the street needing some food. We all need help for something. What can you do to calm a few waves in the ocean of need around us?

What's Your Story?

I just challenged you to try some different strategies for living *beyond belief*, and now I'm going to encourage you with an opportunity. Are you living, striving, or thriving through something? I bet you are. You have a chance, right now, to take ownership of your life—of your own story. Start writing about it. Or, if that seems like a lot, share it with someone. Every single person has a unique story that only they have and no one else.

You are the only person in the world who knows what it means and what it's like to be you—no one else, ever, will have your exact same story. Isn't that wild to think about? You are a totally unique individual, based on your background, experiences, perceptions, personalities, and probably other things. Your story deserves to be shared.

Writing my story has been a journey. Some of the moments early on were hard to write about, and to put myself back in that place, but once I did and got it out there, I could move forward with a renewed sense of confidence. Looking at things from a child's eyes is one thing, but looking back on my experience as an adult, I can understand so much more of my own story.

If you've never thought about how you would begin to share your story, I want to encourage you—it's a neat thing to think about, and can have a lasting impact on you. We can't leave an impact on, or a legacy for, others if we don't share where we've been and what we've learned.

Invitation to Respond

I don't just want to tell you about the hope I have, but I want to share how you can have it, too.

A street-corner preacher had a crowd gathered around him one day at the university I attended for my master's program. In the free speech area of the quad, he had a colorful sign and was warning people that we are all headed down a dark road, and the only way to be saved was to repent and surrender our lives to Jesus. I vividly recall as I weaved my way through the crowd on my way to class, my own Bible in my backpack, a student listening and making fun of this.

The mocker stretched his hands up in the air and exclaimed, "I repent!" as if to show the crowd that nothing would happen and to prove that none of what this preacher said was true. What the young student didn't understand was that repentance starts in our hearts, and we have to gradually stumble through our ego and pride until it can finally reach our lips.

To repent is to recognize and confess we are heading the wrong way, to actively turn around, and head the other direction. We do not just say the words, but we must believe them in our heart and demonstrate the shift with our actions and words. Repentance must be an internal decision, being convicted *beyond belief*, that knowing Jesus is something you just have to do. Other people can help lead you to the ledge, but you're the one who must decide to jump in.

Do you need to repent something? Have you been heading the wrong way and need to change direction? Do you need to confess your desire for a new direction?

God loves as you are, right now, and He wants you to move forward. He wants the best for you, in fact. The point is not just to be happy—a temporary emotion influenced by our external surroundings. God wants you to be able to live *on purpose* in freedom and to live as He has called you—in Faith, Hope, and Love. It will be a tough road at times, but it'll feel good because it'll feel right to walk the path God has called you to walk. In my experience, there's no better feeling than knowing you are following God's call.

I've said a few radical things in this book. Do you have the privilege of suffering for Christ? Maybe God is using your suffering right now for a greater purpose later. Or maybe you've been living one way or thinking some way that just isn't working out for you, and it's causing you heartache and pain. Do you need to repent and set your new direction in life towards Jesus? He might not take away the suffering, but He'll find a way to REDEEM it to work it out for your good.

If so, you can say these words:

"God, I thought I knew what I was doing, but I was wrong. I don't have it all figured out. I realize how much I need you now. I believe Jesus can save me and help me see with new eyes. I repent of my old ways and I want to turn and follow you. Help me do that, God; I can't do it by myself. I invite you into my life, and my heart."

If you prayed that prayer just now, welcome to the family! We call ourselves Christians because we want to follow Jesus Christ. You can message me through my website below if you would like some next steps in your journey of faith.

Conclusion and Send-Off

As I was proofreading and preparing to publish this book, I went back and read my words, thinking, *Wow! This is an amazing message, with so much genuineness, and a thoughtful approach to how the words are laid out.* And it would be a *colossal* mistake to think that I came up with all this stuff myself. (I've tried doing things on my own before, and have totally missed the mark in those moments.) God has been the author of my story, and I would be utterly remiss not to give credit where credit is due.

Growing up, my parents didn't want to share with me how serious my health condition was. They didn't want me to spend my life focused on the edge of the razor on which I was walking. Instead, they wanted me to achieve my potential and experience life unburdened by the lens of medical fragility. The attitude of optimism and gratitude they helped me adopt had a significant part of my becoming who I am today.

Through researching and writing this book, I've learned the gravity of my medical situation and the reality of my symptoms. As a kid, I never cared to really understand all the medical stuff my doctors would talk about at appointments. Now as an adult, where I'm *owning* my conditions, I can see the situation clearly. I'm not taking *accountability* for my brain stem tumor—it's not my fault it's there—but, I'm taking *responsibility* for it, as far as being responsible for what I am going to do about it moving forward. There is no ignoring it (anymore). I'm using the opportunity of a challenge to make an impact on the world, whether that impact is big or small. I don't want to waste the blessing of my brain tumor by ignoring it, I want to celebrate the perspective that God has revealed through this brain tumor.

It has been an incredibly healing process to write this book. To revisit my past and explore some difficult moments has been challenging. But, the important thing is not to *stay* in those moments. We need to focus here, focus now, and focus forward. Yes, those times were hard, the memories are hard, and challenges are still there. But what am I going to do about it *right here* and *right now*, and what will I do moving forward?

My medical journey has shown me how precious life is. Not only should we be grateful for each and every moment we are alive, but our time here is short, and we need to be intentional to make the best use of it before it's gone. None of us know how much longer we will be here to make a difference. Every minute counts.

You have a choice to make, right now. It's not an option to be a bystander. Choose to move forward in hope and faith, or choose to move backward, endlessly spinning wheels. Will you choose faith, hope, and love, or will you choose despair, regret, and envy? We're not getting any younger. Every night you go to sleep is one less day you have on this Earth to make an impact and leave a legacy. I will be making the decision to live *beyond belief*—what about you?

Thank you for the opportunity to share my experiences and thoughts with you. I dearly hope you will take away from this project something of worth, something of value to you in how you live your life. There is always a way to live a better life, and the first step toward reaching that goal is realizing the presence of hope. The choice will make a world of difference.

I used to feel alone and isolated with my medical condition and physical challenges, and I still do sometimes. But, the more I share, the more belonging I feel. And the more belonging we feel, the more we can move forward in this life. We all genuinely belong in this World, and our belonging is found in Jesus.

Epilogue

Having read this book, I want to invite you to one more reading of this poem. And this time, see if it takes on new meaning for you. Feel free to share it or read it out loud.

A Lesson to be Learned

Bad things happen for good reasons.
Although it blinds and divides,
change is in the season.
The time for fun and games is done.
There are rivers to be swum, mountains to be clumb,
valleys to be crossed, and battles to be won.

Boom! The lightning screams as you're shocked out of sleep.
There are no clouds in the sky. There is no rain falling down.
The slope you descend becomes steep.
You tumble past the trees, *whish* and *whoosh*!
Past the trees standing so stably with their deep roots,
you land with a *thump*, dazed and confused.

Dazed and confused, you glance around,
attempt to get your bearings,
but then fail with a frown.
It is too dark to see, too much to bear.

A prickly tingle goes up your back
and you realize you can't go anywhere.

Lost and lonely, you sweat in desperation.
If only you knew which way to go,
which way to face, or your general location
you might find help; you might become found.
But then you remember the creeping darkness,
and all of your hopes vanish into the ground.

This fall takes you back to a notch in your clock
when dark things reigned in your life
and you couldn't wait for that next *tock*.
You try to remember, "Oh, what did I do?
How did I survive? How did I escape
that moment I was feeling so blue?"

Reaching and grasping, running and roaming,
ducking and diving through the dark stormy gloom,
you stop moving to think, and thank God for remembering!
"How does one deal with stormy situations?"
You batten up the hatches!
And prepare the preparations!

And what do the preparations include?
They include a code to live by,
a God at your side, and an attitude that can-do.
Because what makes it easy to feel lost in defeat?
Ignorance, doubt, fear, stress,
and a lonely feeling with no one to greet.

Goodness keeps your mind at ease,

as your instincts say to hide and flee.
Self-control brings you to peace
as your gut feeling shouts, "Panic! Cry!"
Perseverance makes you strong at heart
as the world tells you just to lay down and die.

But wait! What's that at your feet?
As you fall to the floor and feel a great roar
you can maybe, almost, just barely see, though vague and discreet,
a light, far away, as a candle freshly put out.
There is only a faint glow,
but enough to bring hope. You give out a shout!

You wander toward the light,
tripping and falling among the roots and rocks.
Could this bring salvation? It just might!
Faster and faster, brighter and brighter,
the light draws near,
as your feet become lighter.

"Freedom!" you exclaim as you enter a meadow
with bright sunshine falling over where the green grass grows,
where the trees grow tall and the blue waters flow.
Beauty, magnificence, awe, and splendor;
where did this come from?
You look around and ponder in wonder.

Surely, this place is better than before.
Though the tumble down was long and dark,
you're beginning to be grateful, more and more
for the dark road you were forced to go down,
for, eventually, it led to something good.

Though it had you scared stiff, you came to be found.

Found! As the light becomes day
and the day shines so bright,
you wonder how you ever found the way
out of that dark and lonely place,
where bad things happen
and evil shows its face.

There is no mountain without a valley.
There is no rise without a fall.
Look around at the gloom, and think of how it could be.
It could be peaceful, a place that's serene.
Like coming to a breathtaking meadow from the empty dark,
we must only have faith in what is unseen.

And stay holding on, just a little longer, we must.
Before our bones turn to ashes
or our dreams start to rust.
For if we sustain darkness and persevere through the test,
we just might find the light,
and discover our journey was for the best.

But do not go unarmed; do not go alone!
For long is the journey
and dark is the road.
Do not trust appearances; you are only half.
There is another you must take;
He bears a rod and staff.

His rod and staff will comfort you
as the darkness creeps and leads to folly.

Some of his strength He will imbue
if only you declare and claim.
You will find joy in the journey
and, in the painful, not so much pain.

Will you be lost in the forest and get out on your own?
Maybe. But if the present reflects the past,
then your chances are blown.
So choose your side! Take the dare!
But if you do, make sure you do.
Not for me, but for you. Anytime! Anywhere!

Review Inquiry

Hey, it's Kyle here.

I hope you've enjoyed reading *Beyond Belief*, finding it helpful, enlightening, inspiring, and fun. Your time is valuable, and you've chosen to spend some of it reading this book. Thank you, I appreciate your commitment! I'd like to ask you to do one more thing, if I may:

Would you consider giving this book a rating wherever you bought it? Online book stores are more likely to promote a book when they feel good about its content, and reader reviews are a great barometer for a book's quality.

So please go to the website of wherever you bought the book, search for my name and the book title, and leave a review. If able, perhaps consider adding a picture of you holding the book. That increases the likelihood your review will be accepted!

Many thanks in advance,
Kyle Campbell

Will You Share the Love?

Get this book for a friend, associate, or family member!

If you have found this book valuable and know others who would find it useful, consider buying them a copy as a gift. Special bulk discounts are available if you would like your whole team or organization to benefit from reading this. Just contact Kyle.BeyondBelief@gmail.com to inquire.

Would You Like Kyle to Speak to Your Organization or Group?

Book Kyle Now!

Kyle accepts a limited number of speaking and training engagements each year. To learn how you can bring his message to your organization, committee, congregation, or group, email Kyle.BeyondBelief@gmail.com.

About the Author

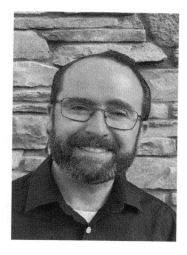

Diagnosed with an inoperable brain stem tumor at age five, Kyle's life has been full of twists and turns. Even after radiation therapy and lots of doctor visits, he still experiences the effects of his brain stem tumor daily. Now, 30 years after his diagnosis and far from the "failure to thrive" he had once been described as exhibiting in his medical reports, Kyle has realized how precious life really is, how we cannot do it on our own, and how important it is to live on purpose with Faith, Focus, and Flexibility.

Kyle has earned a bachelor's degree in philosophy from Cal Poly State University, San Luis Obispo, as well as a master's degree in rehabilitation counseling from California State University, Fresno. He has been the recipient of multiple awards and scholarships, and is nationally recognized as a Certified Rehabilitation Counselor. He has been an editorial assistant, the co-author of a published journal article, and he is excited to share the lessons, perspectives, and active faith that come from living with a brain stem tumor.

Kyle Campbell is a Christian, a preacher, a poet, a philosopher, a professor, and an advocate, but some of his favorite identities are husband and father. Born and raised in the Central Valley of

California, Kyle lives in Visalia, California, with his wonderful wife, Lori, two amazing boys, a third boy on the way, and their dog, Macy.

Kyle can be reached at Kyle.BeyondBelief@gmail.com or online at www.KyleBeyondBelief.com.

Made in the USA
Columbia, SC
22 February 2025

54187495R00091